# The 20 Minutes **Keto Diet Cookbook**

How to lose weight and stay healthy long-term
with delicious recipes including
14 Days Weight Loss Plan and Meal Plan

**Nicholas Edwards**

ISBN: 9781693524707

# CONTENTS

CONTENTS

# EXCLUSIVE BONUS!

## Get Keto Audiobook for FREE NOW!*

***The Ultimate Keto Diet Guide 2019-2020:***
***How to Loose weight with Quick and Easy Steps***

SCAN ME

or go to

www.free-keto.co.uk

*Listen free for 30 Days on Audible (for new members only)

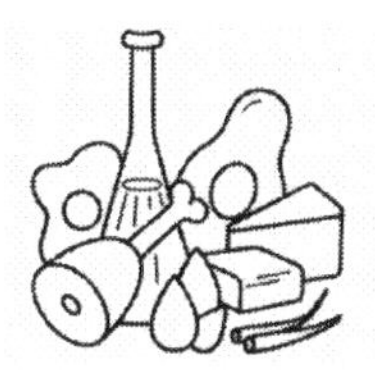

By now everyone has heard the term "keto diet", but what exactly is it and does it really work? Keto, short for ketogenic, is basically a low-carb, high-fat diet, where you eat foods that have a high good fat content and low carbohydrate content. You may have heard of similar diets, like banting for example. Your body's fuel source usually comes from glucose, also known as blood sugar, but we all know that if our blood sugar levels get too high, we run the risk of developing Type 2 Diabetes. Keto actually allows your body to create an alternative fuel source, called ketones. Carbohydrates convert into glucose for energy, but when you reduce your carb intake; your liver begins converting fats into ketones, providing you, especially your brain, with essential energy. When you are following the keto diet, your body changes from running on carbs, to running on fats. Your body is now in a state known as ketosis, and is constantly burning fats for energy. Not only is this great news a bonus for weight watchers, but studies have shown that this food lifestyle can even reverse Type 2 diabetes! Other benefits include staying full for longer, so you stop reaching for that sneaky chocolate for a quick snack. Due to these benefits, many doctors are encouraging patients to try their hand at following the keto diet.

There are a few different styles of the keto diet, aimed at different types of people. The Cycilcal and Targeted Keto Diets are mostly utilized by athletes and bodybuilders, as they are not based on a lifestyle change, but shorter periods of quick dieting. The most common forms of the keto diets are the Standard and the High-Protein Keto Diets. These are the ones that are encouraged by doctors, especially for patients that need to consider their blood sugar levels. The Standard and High-protein keto diets have minute differences, in that the High-protein diet simply incorporates less fat and more protein than the Standard version. The choice of which one suits you best, is entirely up to you. Typically the Standard one uses 75% of fats, 20% of protein and 5% of carbs, whereas the High-protein one uses 60% of fats, 35% of protein and 5% of carbs.

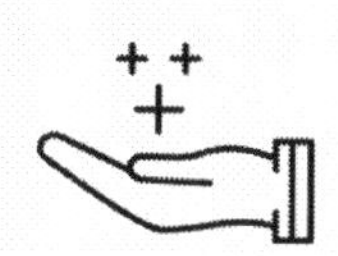

## Losing weight healthily

As we have mentioned, one major benefit to this diet is weight loss and doing it all in a healthy manner. Because your fat-storing hormone (insulin) levels drop, your body becomes a fat-burning machine! Yes, you still have to work at it and dedicate yourself to eating correctly, but what could be better than being slimmer and healthier all at once?!

## Lowers Blood Sugar

Due to the types of food you will eat, the keto diet naturally reduces the blood sugar levels. Some studies have found that the keto diet is the most effective way to control, prevent and even reverse Type 2 diabetes. If you have been diagnosed with Type 2 diabetes, or are even pre-diabetic, you really should consider giving the keto diet a chance.

## Focus and Brain Health

Many people in high pressure jobs use the keto diet to improve their brain health and its ability to keep you focussed and energized. Ketones are a fantastic brain fuel source. Lowering your carbs, helps limit you from having blood sugar spikes. Combining the two improves concentration and keeps you alert.

## Feel Fuller for Longer

The foods you eat on the keto diet are more satisfying due to the high fat content, and they help you feel full for longer periods. Say you have breakfast around 7am, instead of feeling peckish again at 10am, you can actually continue through until lunch time.

## Epilepsy

Keto was actually introduced in the early 1900's, as a successful treatment for epilepsy in children and is still being prescribed today. Epilepsy sufferers who employ the keto diet, report using fewer medicines as a result.

## Blood Pressure and Cholesterol Reductions

Many studies have shown significant improvements in followers of the keto diet, to their triglyceride and cholesterol levels, and their blood pressure. These ailments often are associated with heart problems. Blood pressure is also affected by weight, so the weight loss that comes naturally with keto, is an added bonus to high blood pressure sufferers.

## Acne

Indeed not one you would usually consider, but skin has always seen noticeable improvements when following a low-carb high-fat diet. If you're showing signs of acne or general skin issues, perhaps consider your diet, especially if you're currently eating way too many fast and sugary foods.

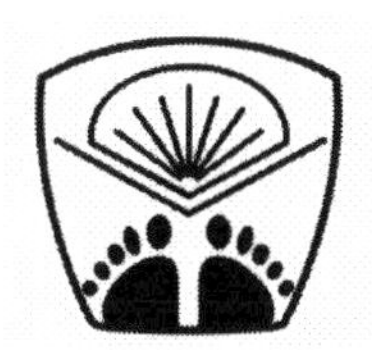

Sick of having to watch what you eat, counting calories and weighing your food, and yet still starving an hour later? Some studies have shown that people following the oft recommended low-fat diet, tend to lose weight, but put it all back on again. Similar studies following keto dieters have found that those dieters have lost considerably more weight. Also they are not starving themselves and have a general improved outlook, both outside with weight loss and inside with improved cholesterol and / or blood sugar. So what's the secret? And how can the keto diet benefit you? Firstly, you need to know which foods you cannot have and eliminate them completely from your diet. It helps to get rid of them from your kitchen entirely, so you're not even tempted. Now, don't be upset when you read this list. Yes, you're going to be giving up a LOT! But, just think about ALL those gains like weight loss (new wardrobe!), healthy brain and heart, more energy, and potentially no more Type 2 diabetes if you're a sufferer.

## Foods to avoid include:

- Sugary foods: This is an obvious one of course, and covers things like soda, fruit juice (even the 100% ones!), cake, ice cream, sweets and candy. Smoothies too, if you haven't made them yourself.

- Starches and grains: Anything made with wheat including pasta, rice, breakfast cereals, bread, etc. An easy way to look at something with grains is to ask if it was made with white flour. If yes, then it's off your list.
- Fruit: Shocker, yes, but not all fruit is off limits. Berries like strawberries, blueberries and even avocados (YES!) are allowed in proportion. Other fruit is off limits because of the carbs in them and they have surprisingly loads.
- Beans and legumes: Peas, beans, chickpeas, etc. Note that peanuts are included in this section, as they are actually legumes and not nuts.
- Root vegetables: Too many carbs in potatoes, carrots, yams and the like.
- Diet / low-fat / sugar-free products: Don't be fooled! These products are highly processed and often high in sugar alternatives and carbs. These can have an adverse affect on your ketone levels and make it harder for you to reach ketosis.
- Sauces and condiments: Mostly contain lots of sugar and bad fats.
- Bad fats: These are things like cooking oil (sunflower, canola, vegetable), margarine and mayonnaise.
- Alcohol: Again, too many carbs. If you want to lose that beer belly, you have to get rid of the beer!

### Foods you're allowed to eat, EAT AND EAT SOME MORE!

- Meat: All meat! Beef, chicken, pork, fish, lamb, rabbit, and more! YES! Bring on that steak!
- Leafy Greens and above-ground vegetables: kale, lettuce, cauliflower. If you do not have to dig it up to eat it, you can eat it!
- Dairy with high-fat content: whole milk, hard cheese, fresh cream, eggs. Skip that 2% and go for the full cream milk!
- Seeds and nuts: cashews, macadamias, sunflower seeds, chia seeds. Excellent snackage material here!
- Berries: Strawberries, raspberries, blueberries, and the best berry of all: the Avocado!
- Sweeteners: Sugar alternatives include erythritol, stevia (which is found in some soft drinks now), xylitol and monk fruit. Be warned though, that if you have pets in the house, you are strongly discouraged from using xylitol, as it is lethal for them.
- Other good fats: Olive oil (preferably extra-virgin), coconut oil, high-fat salad dressings, butter, nut butter.
- Condiments: Not all condiments are banned. Salt, pepper, spiced and herbs are allowed.

See, it's not all bad, right? And we all know that when you have to diet, whether to lose a few pounds or just to get healthier, sacrifices have to be made. With keto, all you need to remember is the food must be high in fats, middle-ground in proteins, and low in carbohydrates. If you're planning on using the Standard keto version, make your per day nutrient intake around 70% high-fat, 25% protein and the remaining 5% carbs. Lowering your carbohydrate intake will improve overall results. Proteins should always been eaten as needed, and the fats filling in all the gaps for the remainder of your day. With weight loss, it's a good trick to note your total carbohydrates and your net carbohydrates. To calculate your net carbs, simply take the total carbs of an item and subtract the total fiber. It is recommended that total carbs per day are kept below 35g and net carbs, ideally, below 20g per day.

In the beginning of getting used to this new lifestyle, you may find yourself getting hungry during the day. Snacking on nuts, seeds, or even some peanut butter should help keep the temptations away. Bear in mind that snacking can slow down your weight loss. If you're weighing yourself periodically and notice very little has changed, go through your day and see how much snacking you have done and decide to either increase the size of a meal, or stop snacking cold turkey.

## Reaching Ketosis

To get the maximum out of the keto diet and all that fat burning going, you need to reach the ketosis stage. Achieving this is quite straightforward, but can seem complicated, so here's a simplified list to get you going:

1. **Limit your carb intake**: Limit all carbs, both total and net carbs. Keeping them below the 35g (total carbs) and 25g (net carbs) recommended limits, will help you to get to the ketosis stage faster.
2. **Limit your protein intake**: Eating too much protein can cause lower levels of ketosis. For weight loss, you ideally need to eat between 0.6g – 0.8g of proteins per pound lean body mass.
3. **Don't stress about fat!** Eating fats is the main source of energy on the keto diet, so ensure you're getting enough. Do not starve yourself!
4. **Drink plenty of water!** Staying hydrated is vital to your body and helps control any hunger pangs too. Try to drink about 2 liters / 0.5 gallons of water per day.
5. **Snacking:** Limit the snacking as it can slow down the process. It also reduces the number of insulin spikes, which elevates your blood sugar levels.

6. **Consider fasting:** A good tool to increase ketone levels is to fast intermittently. This in no way means starving yourself, in the traditional sense of fasting, but simply cutting out a meal here or there. Note thought that fasting is not for everyone, so if you can't, don't.
7. **Exercise:** ah the dreaded exercise. We know that getting exercise is good for us, but not all of us are cut out for going to the gym. If you prefer a more sedentary exercise regime, add in a short walk to help the ketosis along.
8. **Become a label reader:** Some products are designed to catch your eye, as being beneficial to the dieter. This is NOT always the case. Be sure to read the labels carefully and you will be surprised at how many hidden carbs are in so-called diet-friendly products.

## Are you in Ketosis?

There are various products on offer, that can tell you if you're in the ketosis stage, but most of them are expensive and just inaccurate. The following list of things should give you a good indication of whether you are in ketosis:

1. **Needing to urinate more:** The keto diet naturally makes you want to use the bathroom more often.
2. **Dry Mouth:** The more you wee, the more you will get thirsty. Ensure you're drinking plenty of water.

3. **Bad breath:** Not a pleasant thought or what anyone would want to experience. The good thing is that this does not last forever. Just keep some sugar-free (check the labels!) gum nearby, in case you're concerned.
4. **Limited hunger and Energy Boosts:** Once you get into ketosis, you may notice that you can survive longer between meals and have more energy.

## The Keto Flu

While the keto diet is safe for the majority of people, there are some undesirable side effects. We've already mentioned the bad breath, but the one you need to be on the lookout for is the keto flu, also known as carb flu. The symptoms of keto flu can feel similar to actual flu, but are caused by the body trying to adapt to the new eating lifestyle. The drastic reduction of carbohydrate intake shocks your body into withdrawal, because it is now burning ketones instead of glucose for energy.

Symptoms differ from person to person, with varying degrees, but can include any of the following:

- Weakness
- Constipation
- Diarrhoea
- Headaches
- Nausea
- Irritability
- Dizziness
- Muscle cramps and / or soreness
- Vomiting
- Stomach pains
- Inability to concentrate
- Craving for sugar or sugary foods.
- Insomnia

Symptoms usually last for about a week, but can last longer for some people. It's important to know about keto flu and understand what's happening to you, so you don't give up, just as you're getting started. Fortunately, once you recognise that you have keto flu, there are ways to help you get through this miserable period.

1. **Stay hydrated:** Drink plenty of water.
2. **Don't overdo the exercise:** Your body is adapting itself to a new lifestyle, so why punish it even more with exercise? Yes, exercise is important, but during keto-flu, you need to rest.
3. **Restore electrolytes:** The keto diet restricts food items that are high in things like potassium, and magnesium, so try to eat more green leafy veg or avos.
4. **Sleep:** The most common ailment experienced by new keto dieters, is fatigue, which results in irritability. Try limiting your caffeine, or have a warm bath with some lavender bath bombs.
5. **Eat plenty Fats:** Starting on the keto diet will result in cravings for naughty foods. But if you remain strict and eat enough fats, you will keep feeling satisfied and the cravings will disappear.

# BREAKFAST

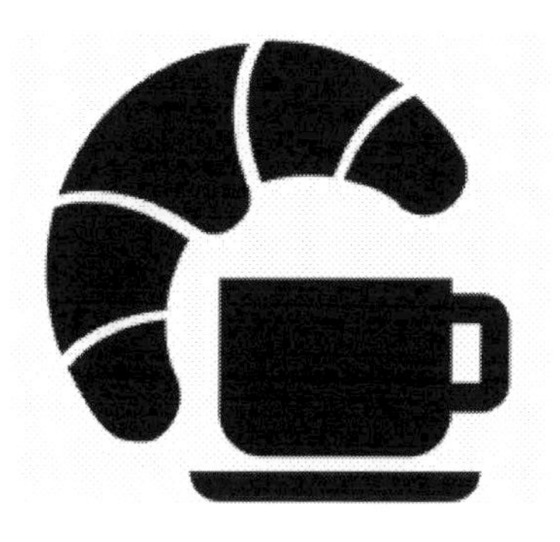

**Serves: 4** kCal: 421 | Carbs: 6.9g | Fat: 27.51g | Protein: 33.53g

## Ingredients

### Waffles

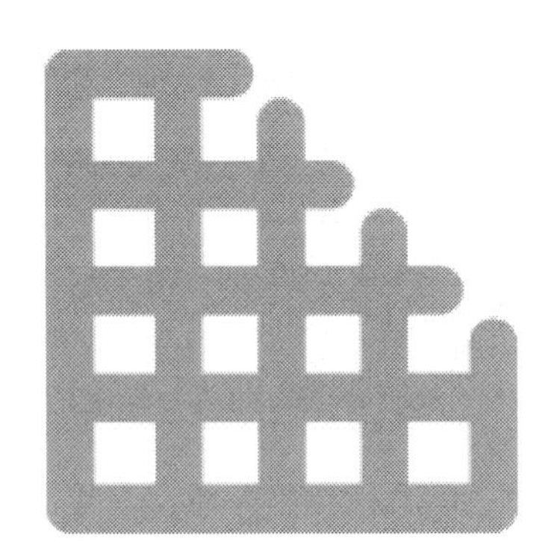

- 2 tablespoons / 28.3g of melted butter
- 3 large eggs, separate the yolks and whites
- ¼ cup / 59ml of milk
- 1 cup / 130gr almond flour
- ½ teaspoon / 2½ gr of salt
- 1 teaspoon/ 5ml of vanilla
- 1 tablespoon / 14gr of erythritol

### Chicken

- 1 cup / 240ml of buttermilk
- 2 medium-sized chicken breast fillets
- 1 large egg
- 1 tablespoon / 14gr olive oil for frying
- Salt and pepper for taste
- 1 teaspoon / 5gr of paprika
- ¼ teaspoon / 2gr of cayenne powder

## Directions

| | |
|---|---|
| **1.** | The night before, cut your chicken breast fillets in half, lengthwise. Cut them again, lengthwise, so you get 4 chicken strips. Soak them in the buttermilk overnight. |
| **2.** | The following morning, season the soaked chicken with the salt, pepper, paprika and cayenne. |
| **3.** | Preheat the oven to 350ºF / 180ºC and preheat your waffle maker. |
| **4.** | In a mixing bowl, beat the 1 large egg. |
| **5.** | In another mixing bowl, mix the almond flour with salt and pepper. |
| **6.** | Place each chicken strip into the flour mixture, coating each side. |
| **7.** | Now coat each chicken strip with the beaten egg, and the flour again, so there are two crumb layers. |
| **8.** | Heat the olive oil in a skillet and quickly add the chicken, cooking each side of the chicken until they are browned. |
| **9.** | Place the chicken strips onto a baking sheet, cover with some foil and bake in the oven for 15 minutes. |
| **10.** | In another mixing bowl, whisk the egg yolks, erythritol, melted butter and vanilla together well. |
| **11.** | Add the almond flour and some salt and whisk again until there are no more lumps. |
| **12.** | With a hand mixer, beat the egg whites until they form stiff peaks. |
| **13.** | Very carefully, adding a small portion at a time, fold the egg whites into the batter. |
| **14.** | Spray some cooking spray on the waffle maker and add □ cup / 79ml portions to it. Cook each waffle for about 5 to 6 minutes until browned. |
| **15.** | Stack the waffle and chicken into a sandwich, keeping the pieces together with a toothpick, and serve. |
| **16.** | You can add option extras like bacon or sugar-free syrup |

**Serves: 4** kCal: 887.68 | Carbs: 8.2g | Fat: 75.4g | Protein: 40.95g

## Ingredients

- 1 pound / 450gr of beef sirloin
- ¼ cup/ 59ml of soy sauce
- 2 tablespoons / 30ml of Calamansi juice*
- 6medium-sized garlic cloves, minced
- 3 teaspoons/ 14gr of garlic powder
- 1 tablespoon / 14gr of granulated eythritol
- 1 cup / 128gr of coconut oil
- 1 pound / 455gr of cauliflower rice
- 4 large eggs
- Salt and pepper

## Directions

| | |
|---|---|
| **1.** | In a mixing bowl, combine the soya sauce, Calamansi juice, garlic (leave some for later), garlic powder (leave some for later), erythritol, salt and pepper together. Mix until the salt and erythritol are completely dissolved. |
| **2.** | Put the beef sirloin into a Ziploc bag and pour the marinade over the beef, in the bag. Seal the bag and place in the fridge overnight. |
| **3.** | The following day, take the meat out of the bag. |
| **4.** | Coat a frying pan with some of the coconut oil and heat. Add the beef to the pan and fry until all the liquid is almost absorbed. Turn the meat repeatedly. |
| **5.** | Remove the beef and allow to cool, before slicing into strips. |
| **6.** | Add the remaining coconut oil and minced garlic, garlic powder and some salt to the pan and sauté until it is aromatic. |
| **7.** | Toss in the cauliflower rice and coat evenly, cooking until the rice is tender |
| **8.** | In a separate frying pan, fry the eggs as desired. |
| **9.** | Once cooked, layer a bowl with the cauliflower rice, then the beef, top with the eggs and serve. |
| **10.** | *Calamansi juice is a Filipino variation of lemonade. |

# BLUEBERRY PANCAKE BITES

**Serves: 6** kCal: 174.77 | Carbs: 7.07g | Fat: 13.27g | Protein: 6.52g

## Ingredients

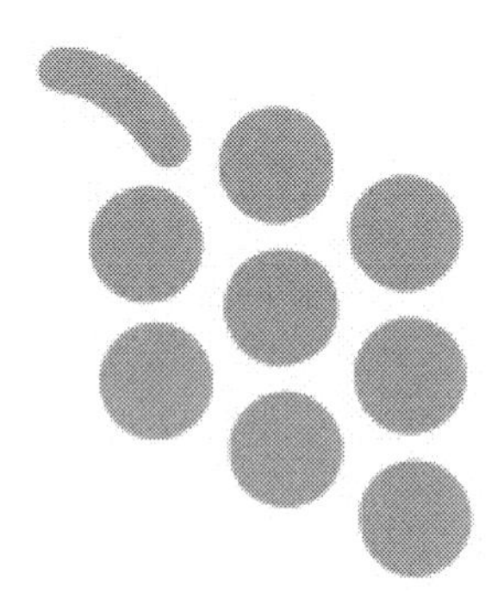

- 4 large eggs
- ¼ cup / 85gr of erythritol
- ½ teaspoon / 2½ ml of vanilla extract
- ½ cup / 170gr of coconut flour
- ¼ cup / 85gr of melted butter
- 1 teaspoon / 5gr of baking powder
- ½ teaspoon / 2½ gr of salt
- ¼ teaspoon / 2gr of cinnamon
- □ cup / 80ml of water
- ½ cup / 170gr of frozen blueberries

## Directions

| | |
|---|---|
| **1.** | Preheat the oven to 325ºF/ 165ºC. |
| **2.** | Greaseproof a muffin tin extremely well, as the mixture is very sticky. |
| **3.** | In a blender, mix the eggs, erythritol, and vanilla extract together. |
| **4.** | To the mixture, add the coconut flour, melted butter, baking powder, salt and cinnamon and blend again, until smooth. |
| **5.** | Allow the mixture to rest for a few minutes to thicken up. |
| **6.** | Add the water in □ portions to the mixture, blending each time. |
| **7.** | Blend until the mixture is scoopable, but not pourable. |
| **8.** | Fill each muffin spot with the mixture, and top off with some blueberries, pushing them into the mixture. |
| **9.** | Bake for 25 minutes. To test if they are ready, stick a toothpick into the center of one, and if it comes out clean, it's ready. If not, bake for a few mins more, checking all the time. |
| **10.** | Serve with some sugar-free syrup. |

# STUFFED PEPPERS

**Serves: 4** kCal: 245.5 | Carbs: 5.97g | Fat: 16.28g | Protein: 17.84g

## Ingredients

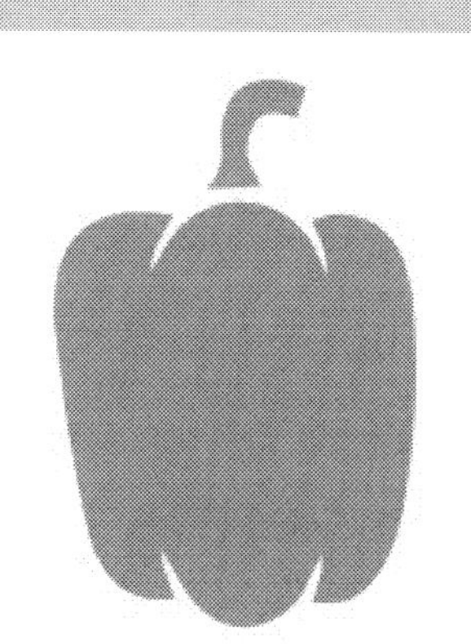

- 4 large eggs
- 2medium-sized bell peppers.
- ½ cup 170gr of ricotta cheese
- ½ cup / 170gr of shredded mozzarella
- ½ cup / 170gr of parmesan cheese, grated
- 1 teaspoon / 5gr of garlic powder
- ¼ teaspoon / 2gr of dried parsley
- ¼ cup / 85gr of baby spinach leaves
- 2 tablespoons / 28gr of extra parmesan cheese for garnishing

## Directions

| | |
|---|---|
| 1. | Preheat the oven to 375ºF / 190ºC. |
| 2. | Slice the peppers in equal halves and remove the seeds. |
| 3. | In a blender/food processor, add the cheeses, eggs, garlic powder and parsley and mix well. |
| 4. | Pour the mixture into each pepper half to just below the top. Add some spinach leaves and push them into the mixture with a fork. |
| 5. | Prepare a baking sheet, place the filled pepper halves onto the baking sheet and cover with foil. |
| 6. | Bake for about 35 – 45 minutes, or until the egg has set. |
| 7. | Sprinkle with the remaining parmesan cheese and grill for a further 3 – 5 minutes until the tops brown. |

# SPICY EGGS AND CHEESY HASH

**Serves: 3** kCal: 248 | Carbs: 5.77g | Fat: 18.14g | Protein: 12.57g

## Ingredients

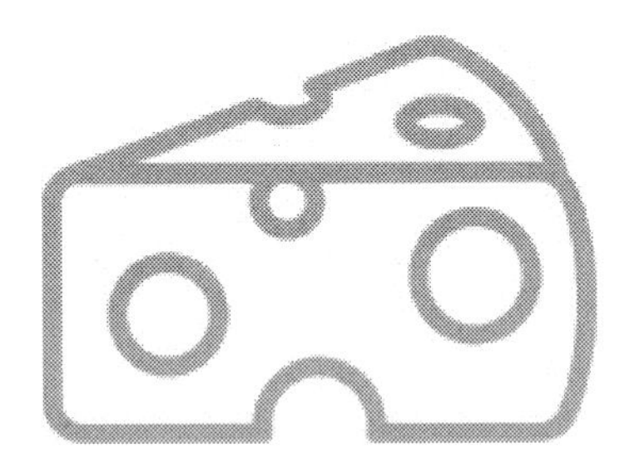

- 5oz / 142gr of diced zucchini
- 6oz / 170gr of chopped cauliflower
- ½ medium-sized diced red bell-pepper
- 1 tablespoon / 15gr of melted coconut oil
- 1 teaspoon / 5gr of paprika
- 1 teaspoon / 5gr of onion powder
- ½ teaspoon / 2½ gr of garlic powder
- ¼ cup / 85gr of Mexican blend shredded cheese
- ½ of a medium-sized avocado, sliced
- 3 large eggs
- 3 tablespoons / 42gr of cotija cheese
- 2 teaspoons / 10gr of Tajin seasoning
- 1 tablespoon/ 5gr of sliced jalapeno (optional)

## Directions

| | |
|---|---|
| **1.** | Preheat the oven to 400ºF / 205ºC. |
| **2.** | Prepare a baking sheet with foil. |
| **3.** | Spread in an even layer, the zucchini, cauliflower and red pepper and drizzle with the coconut oil. |
| **4.** | Sprinkle on the veg, the onion powder, garlic and paprika and toss to coat everything well. Spread into a layer again. |
| **5.** | Bake for around 10 – 15 mins until the veg begins to brown. |
| **6.** | Take the veg out the oven and sprinkle the shredded Mexican cheese over the top. |
| **7.** | Arrange the avo slices amongst the roasted veg and crack the 3 eggs into spaces in between. |
| **8.** | Bake for a further 10 mins until the eggs are done. |
| **9.** | Garnish with the cotija cheese, Tajin seasoning and optional jala-peno and serve. |

# FAUX-TATOE BUBBLE AND SQUEAK

**Serves: 3** kCal: 332.67 | Carbs: 8.6g | Fat: 28.11g | Protein: 10.65g

## Ingredients

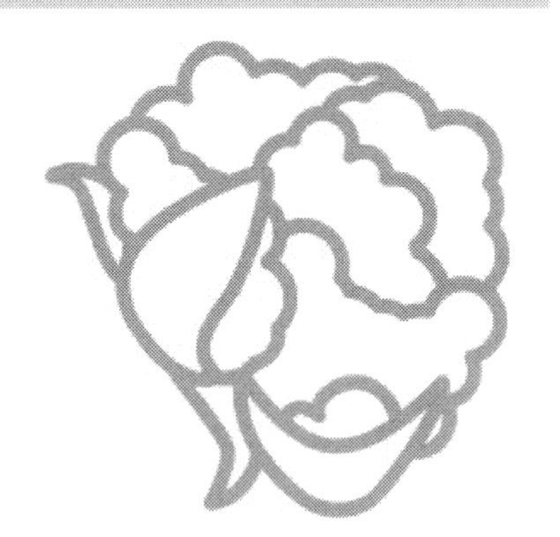

### Mashed Cauliflower

- ½ of a medium-sized cauliflower, cut into florets
- 2 tablespoons / 28gr heavy whipping cream
- 1 tablespoon/ 15gr butter
- Salt and pepper to taste

### Bubble and Squeak

- 3 bacon slices, diced
- 1 tablespoon/ 15gr of butter
- ¼ of a medium-sized onion, diced
- 1½oz / 50gr of leek,sliced
- 1 green onion, sliced
- 1½oz / 50gr of Brussels sprouts, chopped
- ¼ cup / 85gr of mozzarella
- ¼ cup / 85gr of parmesan cheese
- 2 tablespoons / 28gr of duck fat
- 1 teaspoon / 5gr minced garlic

## Directions

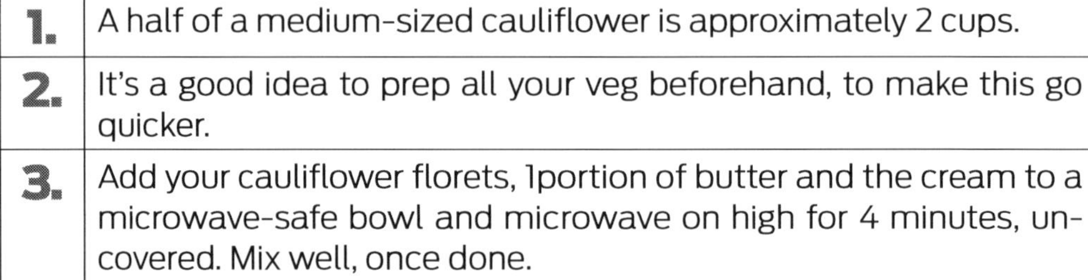

| | |
|---|---|
| 1. | A half of a medium-sized cauliflower is approximately 2 cups. |
| 2. | It's a good idea to prep all your veg beforehand, to make this go quicker. |
| 3. | Add your cauliflower florets, 1portion of butter and the cream to a microwave-safe bowl and microwave on high for 4 minutes, uncovered. Mix well, once done. |
| 4. | Microwave for 4 minutes more, until the cauliflower is soft. Season with salt and pepper. |

| | |
|---|---|
| **5.** | Using a stick blender, blend the cauliflower mixture until thick and creamy. While it's still hot, add the mozzarella so it melts. Set aside to cool down. |
| **6.** | Using a pan on a medium-high heat, cook your bacon until crispy and the fat is rendered out. |
| **7.** | Place the bacon on a paper towel. |
| **8.** | Add the 2nd portion of butter to the bacon fat in the pan, along with the garlic, and cook for a minute on a medium heat. |
| **9.** | Add the onion and cook until the onion is semi-transparent. |
| **10.** | Add the leeks and Brussels sprouts and cook until soft. About 5 – 10 mins. |
| **11.** | Add the green onion and cook for another minute. |
| **12.** | Take off the heat and allow to cool. |
| **13.** | Add the bacon to the veggie mix and then add the mashed cauliflower. Taste and season if required. |
| **14.** | Combine the veggies and mashed cauliflower well. |
| **15.** | Using a separate pan, heated over a medium heat, add the duck fat. |
| **16.** | Once it's melted, place egg rings into the pan and add some parmesan cheese inside the rings. |
| **17.** | Add the cauliflower veggie mix to each ring and sprinkle some more parmesan over the top. |
| **18.** | Warm each "pattie" through and flip, cooking until a crust forms. |
| **19.** | Don't let them get too hot, as the mixture may run. |

# BACON BAGELS

**Serves: 3** kCal: 605.67 | Carbs: 5.76g | Fat: 50.29g | Protein: 30.13g

## Ingredients

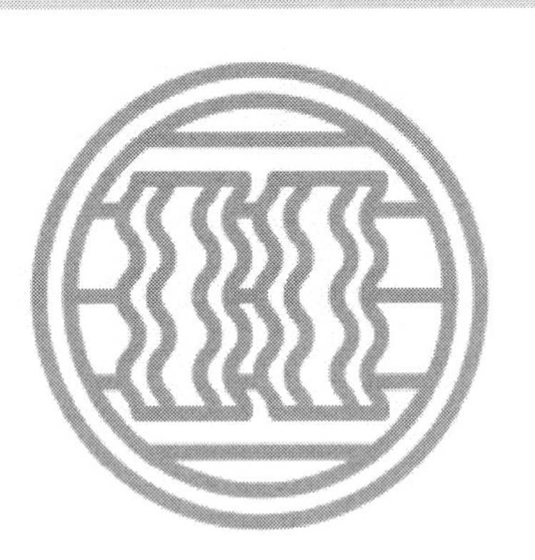

### Bagels

- ¾ cup / 98gr almond flour
- 1 teaspoon / 5gr xanthan gum
- 1 large egg
- 1½ cups / 510gr grated mozzarella cheese
- 2 tablespoons / 28gr cream cheese

### Toppings

- 1 tablespoon / 15gr melted butter
- Some sesame seeds for taste

### Fillings

- 2 tablespoons / 28gr pesto
- 2 tablespoons / 28gr cream cheese
- 1 cup / 340gr arugula leaves
- 6 slices of cooked bacon

## Directions

| | |
|---|---|
| 1. | Preheat the oven to 390ºF / 200ºC. |
| 2. | Mix together the almond flour and the xanthan gum. |
| 3. | Add the egg and mix until well combined, to look like a doughy ball. |
| 4. | Put a pot on a medium-low heat and slowly melt the cream cheese and mozzarella together. Take off the heat once melted. |
| 5. | Add the melted cheese mixture to the flour mixture and knead well. Persist through until is it well combined. |
| 6. | It's crucial that the xanthan gum is combined very well into the cheese mixture. If the dough gets tough, microwave for a few seconds to warm it and knead again until it resembles dough. |
| 7. | Divide the dough into 3 equal pieces and roll into logs. |
| 8. | Make the logs into circles by joining the ends together and place on a greased baking tray. |
| 9. | Melt the butter and brush the bagel tops and sprinkle on the sesame seeds. |
| 10. | Bake the bagels for around 18 minutes, until the tops are a golden brown. Keep an eye on them, as every oven is different. |
| 11. | Cook your bacon as desired. |
| 12. | Slice your bagels in half, spread some cream cheese, and add some pesto, arugula and bacon. |

# RICOTTA AND BLUEBERRY PANCAKES

**Serves: 5** kCal: 311.4 | Carbs: 5.78g | Fat: 22.61g | Protein: 15.25g

## Ingredients

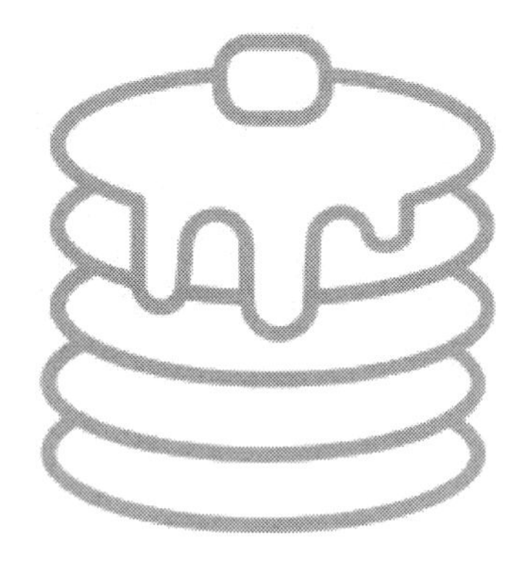

- 3 large eggs
- ¾ cup / 200gr of ricotta cheese
- ½ teaspoon / 2½ gr of vanilla extract
- ¼ cup / 60ml of unsweetened vanilla almond milk
- 1 cup / 130gr of almond flour
- ½ cup / 65gr of golden flaxseed meal
- ¼ teaspoon / 2gr of salt
- 1 teaspoon / 5gr of baking powder
- ¼ teaspoon / 2gr of stevia
- ¼ cup / 85gr of blueberries

## Directions

| | |
|---|---|
| 1. | Preheat a skillet on a medium heat. |
| 2. | Blend the eggs, ricotta cheese, vanilla extract and almond milk together. |
| 3. | In a separate mixing bowl, mix the almond flour, flaxseed meal, salt, baking powder and stevia together. |
| 4. | Slowly add the dry Ingredients to the wet Ingredients and blend together until smooth. |
| 5. | Melt the butter in the skillet. |
| 6. | Using a 2 tablespoon measurement, scoop the batter and pour into the skillet. |
| 7. | Add 3-4 blueberries to each scoop/pancake. |
| 8. | When lightly browned on one side, flip and do the other side. |
| 9. | Serve with sugar-free syrup or extra berries |

# CHORIZO BAKED EGGS

**Serves: 4** kCal: 321 | Carbs: 2.02g | Fat: 27.31g | Protein: 15.57g

## Ingredients

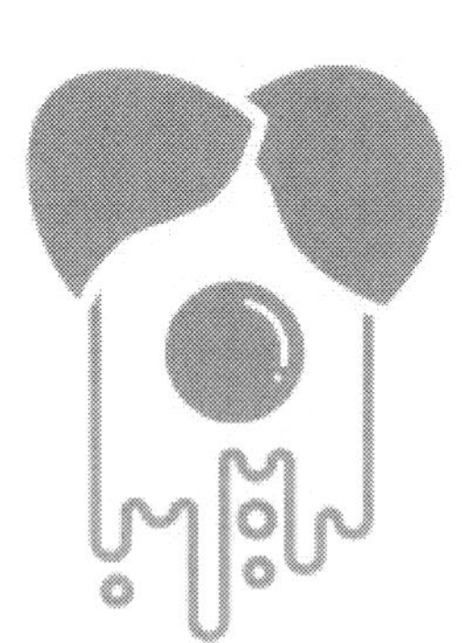

- 5 large eggs
- 2oz / 56gr of Mexican-style pork chorizo
- 2 tablespoons / 28gr of butter
- Salt and pepper for tasting
- □ cup / 85gr of shredded pepper jack cheese
- 1 medium-sized avocado
- 2 tablespoons / 28gr of sour cream
- 2 tablespoons / 28gr of chopped cilantro for some optional garnish

## Directions

| | |
|---|---|
| **1.** | Preheat the oven to 400ºF / 205ºC. |
| **2.** | Over a medium heat, preheat an oven-safe skillet. |
| **3.** | Remove the chorizo casings and add the meat to the skillet. Fry until cooked and allow to drain on some paper towels. |
| **4.** | Add the butter to the skillet and allow it to melt. Ensure the whole pan is evenly coated with butter. Take the pan off the heat and place on a heat-proof surface. |
| **5.** | Into the buttered pan, crack 3 of the eggs and sprinkle with some salt and pepper. |
| **6.** | Add some chorizo on top of the eggs and sprinkle cheese evenly over the whole dish. |
| **7.** | Put the pan into the oven for 15 – 20 minutes, until you see the cheese start to bubble. |
| **8.** | Bake for shorter periods if you prefer a more runny egg yolk. |
| **9.** | Serve warm with the avo, sour cream and optional cilantro. |

# EGGS BENEDICT CASSEROLE

**Serves: 8** kCal: 483 | Carbs: 2.78g | Fat: 33.41g | Protein: 18.54g

## Ingredients

- 12 large eggs
- 8oz / 227gr of unsalted butter
- 19½oz / 553gr of peeled eggplant
- 1lb / 450gr of pre-cooked ham
- 6 large egg yolks
- ¼ cup / 60ml of heavy whipping cream
- Salt and pepper for tasting
- 2 tablespoons / 30ml of white vinegar
- ¼ teaspoon / 2gr of crushed peppercorns
- 1 tablespoon / 15gr of water
- Lemon juice for tasting

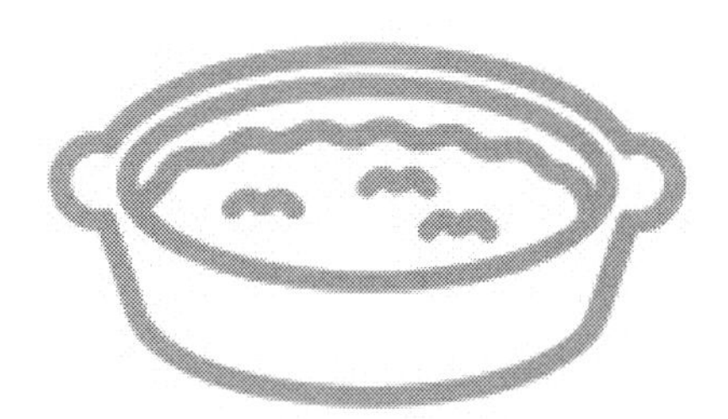

## Directions

| | |
|---|---|
| **1.** | Preheat the oven to 375ºF / 190ºC. |
| **2.** | Over a low heat in a heavy saucepan, melt your butter. |
| **3.** | Once it's melted, you will notice foam rising to the surface. Remove this foam until it stops. |
| **4.** | Carefully pour the melted butter into a heat-proof container, and prevent any solids from going with the butter. |
| **5.** | Wash, chop and dice the eggplant. |
| **6.** | Grease a casserole dish well and add the prepared eggplant. |
| **7.** | Dice the ham and add it on top of the eggplant. |
| **8.** | In a mixing bowl, crack the 12 eggs and season with some salt and pepper |
| **9.** | Add the cream and whisk until well combined. |
| **10.** | Pour the egg mixture over the ham and eggplant. |

| | |
|---|---|
| **11.** | Mix around to make sure everything is well coated with egg mixture. |
| **12.** | Cover the casserole with foil and bake for 30mins. |
| **13.** | Uncover and bake for another 20 – 30 mins, until the egg is cooked. |
| **14.** | While the casserole is in the oven, you can continue with the Hollandaise sauce. |
| **15.** | Make sure your melted butter is still in liquid form and warm. |
| **16.** | Preheat a skillet, add the vinegar and peppercorns and cook until the vinegar has almost evaporated. Add the water. |
| **17.** | You will need a mixing bowl that can fit over a saucepan and be used as a double boiler. |
| **18.** | Transfer the vinegar and peppercorn mixture to this mixing bowl. |
| **19.** | Add the 6 egg yolks to the mixing bowl and whisk everything together. |
| **20.** | Place the mixing bowl over a saucepan of boiling water. |
| **21.** | Lower the heat and whisk until the egg yolks have thickened. |
| **22.** | Remove from the heat and slowly drizzle the melted butter into egg yolk mixture, while whisking. Adding too quickly will break the emulsion, so go slowly. |
| **23.** | Add the lemon juice and some salt to taste. |
| **24.** | If your sauce requires thinning, add 2 – 3 tablespoons of water, one tablespoon at a time, until it reaches desired consistency. |
| **25.** | Your casserole should be done by this point, so go ahead and pour the sauce over the casserole. |
| **26.** | Garnish with whatever you like, such as green onion, or chives and serve. |

**Serves: 1** kCal: 604.8 | Carbs: 9g | Fat: 46.5g | Protein: 34.5g

## Ingredients

### Dressing

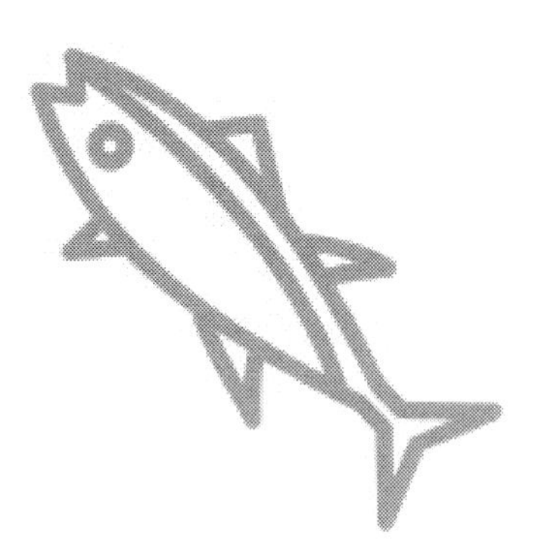

- 1 tablespoon / 15ml of olive oil
- ½ tablespoon / 7½ml of apple cider vinegar
- Salt and pepper for tasting

### Salad

- 4 large iceberg lettuce leaves
- 1 small-sized tomato
- ½ of a small cucumber
- ¼ medium-sized avocado

### Tuna

- 1 can of tuna in oil, drained
- 1½ tablespoons / 23gr of mayonnaise
- 1½ tablespoons / 23gr of full-fat Greek yogurt*
- 1 tablespoon / 15gr of pesto
- 2 teaspoons / 10ml of lemon juice
- Salt for tasting

## Directions

| | |
|---|---|
| 1. | *You may want to substitute the yogurt for more mayo instead. |
| 2. | Add the olive oil, vinegar, salt and pepper to a container with a secure lid. Close the lid and shake to combine everything together. Set aside. |
| 3. | Tear the lettuce leaves and place in a bowl. |
| 4. | Chop up the tomatoes, cucumber, and avo and add to the leaves. |
| 5. | In a separate bowl, mix the tuna, mayo, yogurt, pesto, lemon juice and some salt together. |
| 6. | Add the tuna mixture on top of the salad and drizzle with the dressing. |

# STEAK AND MUSHROOM STROGANOFF

**Serves: 1** kCal: 594.52 | Carbs: 6.9g | Fat: 49g | Protein:33.1g

## Ingredients

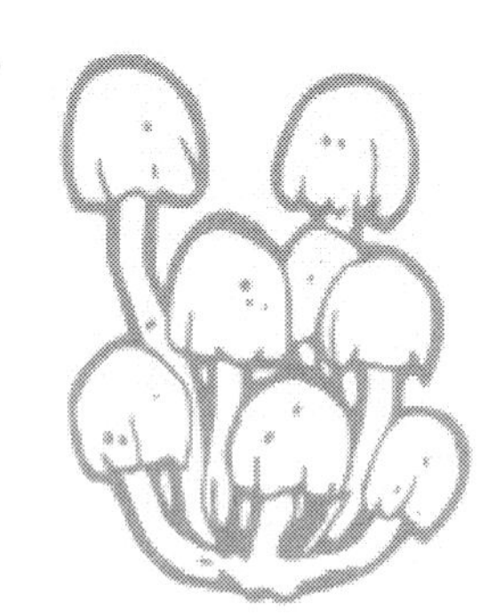

- 1 tablespoon/ 15gr of butter
- Salt and pepper for tasting
- 4oz / 114gr of ribeye steak
- 4oz / 114gr of whole mushrooms, cut into quarters.
- 1 large garlic clove, minced
- 3 tablespoons / 45ml of chicken stock
- 1½ oz / 43gr of cream cheese
- ¼ teaspoon / 2ml of Worcestershire sauce
- ¼ teaspoon/ 2gr of black pepper (for the sauce)
- 1 teaspoon / 5gr of minced parsley

## Directions

| | |
|---|---|
| **1.** | Over a medium-high heat, preheat a skillet and add half of the butter. |
| **2.** | Add the steak to the pan, sprinkle some salt and pepper over the steak and sear it. Set aside. |
| **3.** | Add the remaining butter to the pan and once melted, add the mushrooms and cook until they have softened. |
| **4.** | Lower the heat to low, add the garlic and cook for another minute. |
| **5.** | Add the chicken stock, and using a wooden spoon, scrape the brown bits from the bottom of the pan. This is all the flavour! |
| **6.** | Add the cream cheese, Worcestershire sauce, black pepper and stir together until the cheese has melted. |
| **7.** | Put the steak on a plate, top it off with the stroganoff sauce, garnish with the parsley and serve. |

# CHEESY BEER SOUP

**Serves: 6** kCal: 382.82 | Carbs: 6.87g | Fat: 30.3g | Protein: 17.39g

## Ingredients

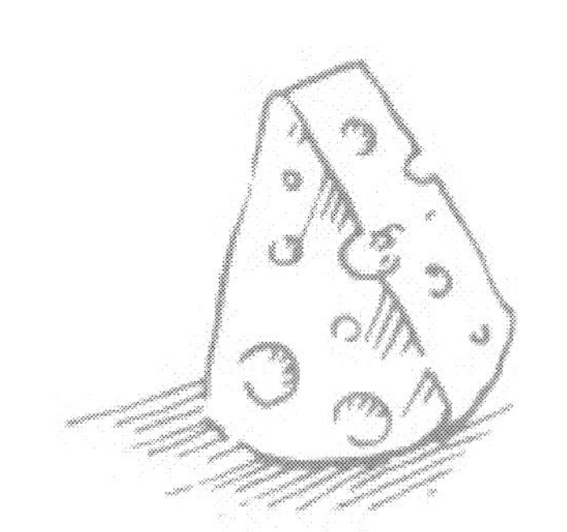

- 3 cups / 705ml of chicken stock
- 1 bottle (12oz)/ 350ml low carb beer
- ½ cup / 120ml heavy whipping cream
- 2 teaspoons / 10gr of xanthan gum
- 6 slices of cooked and diced bacon
- 12oz / 341gr of grated cheddar cheese
- 1tablespoon / 15gr of butter
- ½ cup / 130gr of diced onion
- 2 cloves of minced garlic
- ½ of a small red bell-pepper, diced
- 1 tablespoon / 15ml of Dijon mustard
- 1 teaspoon / 5gr of celery salt
- 1 teaspoon / 5gr of black pepper
- ½ teaspoon / 2½ gr of paprika
- ¼ teaspoon / 2gr of cayenne pepper

## Directions

| | |
|---|---|
| 1. | Get out your stock pot and heat it over a medium heat. |
| 2. | Add the butter and heat it up. |
| 3. | Once it's hot, add the bell-pepper and onion and sauté until they have softened. |
| 4. | Add the garlic and cook until the garlic is aromatic. |
| 5. | Pour in the beer, chicken stock and the heavy cream. |
| 6. | Add the celery salt, black pepper, paprika and cayenne pepper, stirring occasionally while it heats up. |
| 7. | Adding the xanthan gum may start clumping so to prevent that, add a little of the soup to a small bowl. Add the xanathan gum to this and whisk together. Then add that to the main pot of soup. |
| 8. | Continue stirring until the soup thickens |
| 9. | A handful at a time, add the cheese. Allow it to dissolve before adding the next handful. |
| 10. | Pour into serving bowls, add the diced bacon on top and serve. |

**Serves: 4** kCal: 360.25 | Carbs: 1.7g | Fat: 16.76g | Protein: 47.08g

## Ingredients

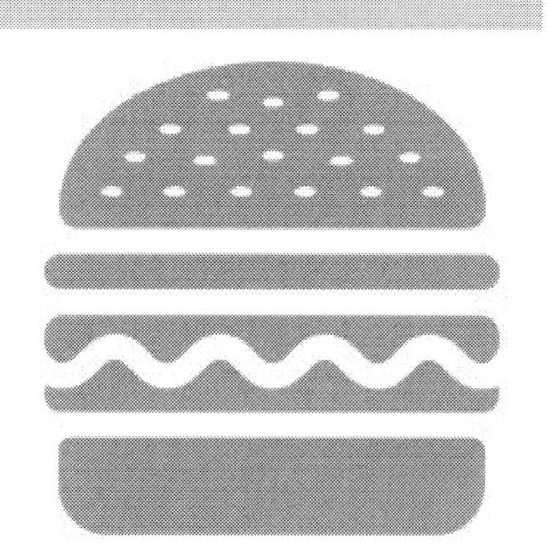

- 1½lb / 680gr freshly caught salmon filets
- 1½ tablespoons / 45gr of mayonnaise
- 1½ tablespoons / 45gr of mustard
- ½ of a small red onion, diced
- 2 tablespoons / 28gr of fresh dill
- 1 celery stalk, diced
- 2 minced garlic cloves
- 2 teaspoons / 10gr of salt
- 1 teaspoon / 5gr of black pepper
- Fresh lemon juice for tasting

## Directions

| | |
|---|---|
| **1.** | You will require some cedar planks that you can find in many grocery stores in the grilling section. They give amazing flavor to your food, so why not give it a go? |
| **2.** | Soak your cedar planks in water, for 2 hours before you start cooking. Make sure you get enough planks for all your salmon burgers. |
| **3.** | Preheat the grill (indirect heat), to around 350ºF / 180ºC. |
| **4.** | Prepare your salmon by removing the skin and any bones. |
| **5.** | Cut into small pieces and add to a food processor. |
| **6.** | Add the mayonnaise, mustard, dill, salt, pepper and the garlic on top of the salmon. |
| **7.** | Pulse the food processor until the salmon becomes like a smooth paste. |
| **8.** | Put everything into a mixing bowl and add the onion and celery. |
| **9.** | Put the soaked planks onto the grill and allow them to warm up. |
| **10.** | Form the salmon mixture into burger shapes. |
| **11.** | Place two burgers on each plank and grill them for about 20 – 35 minutes until the salmon is cooked through. |
| **12.** | Take the planks off the heat, and squeeze some lemon juice on top of the burgers. |
| **13.** | Serve with your favorite toppings. |

**Serves: 10**

kCal: 303.41 | Carbs: 3.29g | Fat: 23.4g | Protein: 18.45g

## Ingredients

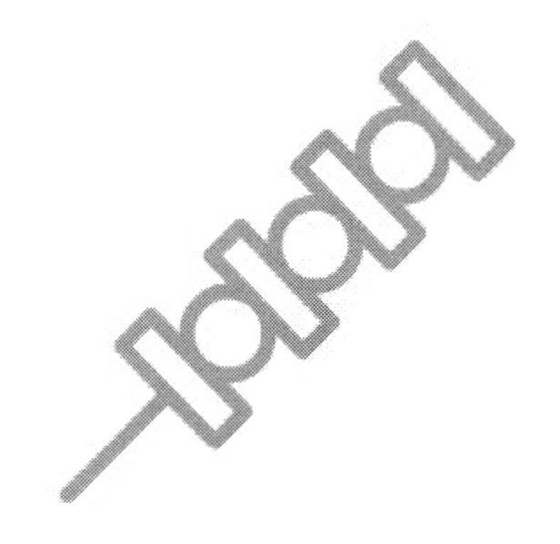

### Kebabs

- 1lb / 455gr of ground beef
- 1 tablespoon/ 15ml of Worcestershire sauce
- ½ teaspoon / 2½gr of salt
- 1 teaspoon / 5gr of black pepper
- 1 teaspoon/ 15gr of dried minced onion
- 6 slices of bacon
- 5 slices of cheddar cheese, cut into quarters
- ½ a head of an iceberg lettuce
- 10 cherry tomatoes
- 20 dill pickle slices

### Dipping Sauce

- ½ cup / 120ml mayonnaise
- 2 tablespoons/ 30ml of sugar-free ketchup
- 1 tablespoon/ 15ml of mustard
- 2 tablespoons/ 28gr of minced onion
- 2 tablespoons/ 28gr of minced dill pickles
- Pickle juice for tasting

## Directions

| | |
|---|---|
| 1. | Preheat the grill at 375ºF / 190ºC. You will need to be able to do direct and indirect grilling. |
| 2. | In a mixing bowl, add the ground beef, Worcestershire sauce, salt, pepper, garlic powder, and dried minced onion and mix together well. |
| 3. | Scoop out and form evenly sized balls. |
| 4. | Flatten them out into a burger shape. |
| 5. | Place a cast iron skillet over the indirect heat and cook the bacon. Not too crispy, as you still need to put it on the skewer. Once cooked, set aside. |
| 6. | Place the skillet back onto the indirect heat and add your burger patties. Cook one side, turn and cook until cooked through. |
| 7. | Move the skillet to the direct heat and sear both sides of the burgers. |
| 8. | Once cooked through, add a slice of cheese to the top of the burgers, and allow to melt. Set aside. |
| 9. | Using large skewers stack the patties, bacon, lettuce, tomatoes, and pickle slices. |
| 10. | Mix the dipping sauce Ingredients together in a bowl and serve with the kebabs. |

**Serves: 1** kCal: 392.17 | Carbs: 6.3g | Fat: 46.49g | Protein: 13.23g

## Ingredients

### For the Filling

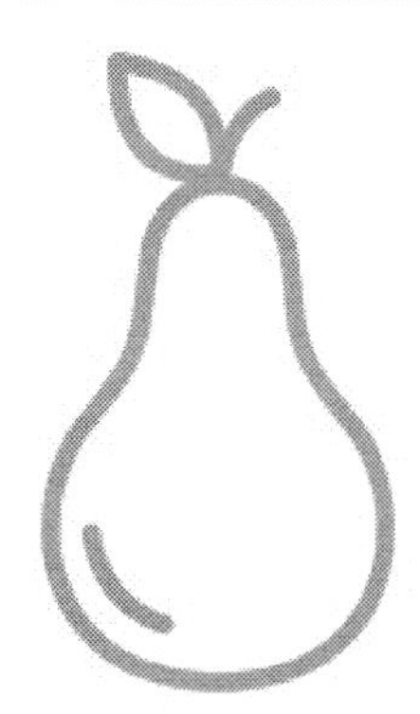

- 7oz / 198gr of cauliflower
- 1 cup / 120gr of raw walnuts
- 1 tablespoon/ 15gr of hulled hemp seeds
- 1 teaspoon/ 5gr of cumin
- 1 teaspoon/ 5grof garlic powder
- 1 teaspoon/ 5grof onion powder
- 2 teaspoons/ 10gr of smoked paprika
- 2teaspoons / 10gr of adobo sauce
- 4tablespoons / 60ml of avocado oil, divided between 2 tablespoons
- 2 tablespoons / 10gr of grated cheddar
- 1 teaspoon / 5gr of salt

### For the Avocado Boats

- ½ cup / 170gr of taco filling
- ½ of a medium-sized avocado
- 1 tablespoon of sour cream
- 1 tablespoon of grated cheddar

## Directions

| | |
|---|---|
| 1. | Divide the cauliflower up into florets and add to a food processor. |
| 2. | Add the walnuts, hemp seeds and seasonings to the food processor. |
| 3. | Pulse until the cauliflower and nuts become like a crumble. |
| 4. | Heat one half of the avocado oil in a skillet, over a medium heat. |
| 5. | Add one half of the "taco meat" (cauliflower) mixture to the skillet, stir well until the nuts are toasted and the cauliflower softens |
| 6. | Add half the adobo sauce to the skillet, folding it into the mixture. Make sure the mixture is browning evenly. |
| 7. | Take off from the heat and fold in the cheese, season with salt and put into a bowl. |
| 8. | Repeat with the rest of the taco filling. |
| 9. | Slice the avo in half, remove the stone. |
| 10. | Scoop a portion of the avo out to make room for the taco filling. |
| 11. | Fill the avo with ½ cup of your prepared taco mixture, top with sour cream and cheddar. |

**Serves: 2**

kCal: 328.55 | Carbs: 6.23g | Fat: 27.85g | Protein: 13.5g

## Ingredients

- 4 slices of bacon
- 2cups / 134gr of kale
- ¼ cup / 35gr of sweet onion
- ½ cup / 60gr of raw walnuts
- 2 teaspoons / 6gr of erythritol
- ½ teaspoon / 2½ ml of maple syrup
- 1 tablespoon/ 15ml of lemon juice

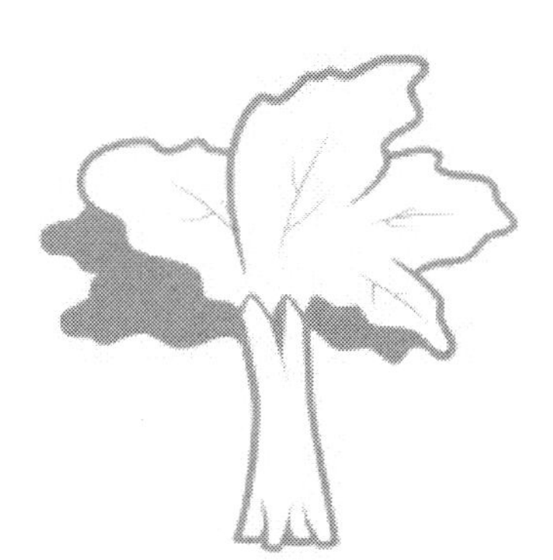

## Directions

| | |
|---|---|
| 1. | Cook the bacon to the desired crispiness. |
| 2. | Place bacon on a plate and allow to cool. |
| 3. | Add the walnuts to the bacon grease in the pan and cook on a medium heat, stirring enough to coat all the nuts. |
| 4. | Cut the kale leaves into bite-sizes and remove the stems. Put into a bowl. |
| 5. | Dice the onion. |
| 6. | Sprinkle the erythritol and maple syrup over the walnuts in the pan. Stir to coat evenly. |
| 7. | Add the onion to the walnuts and sauté until soft and the walnuts have caramelized. |
| 8. | Take the pan off the heat and drizzle some lemon juice over the top. |
| 9. | Cut the bacon strips into smaller bits. |
| 10. | Pour the maple walnut mixture over the kale and toss to coat evenly. |
| 11. | Sprinkle the bacon over the top and serve. |

**Serves: 3**

kCal: 333.63 | Carbs: 2.5g | Fat: 31.73g | Protein: 14.77g

## Ingredients

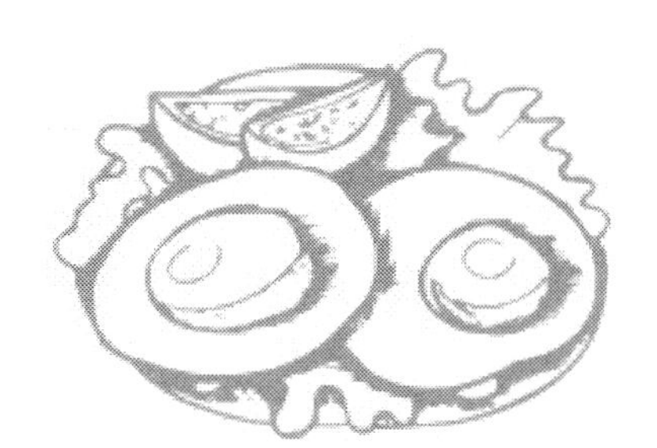

- 3 strips of bacon
- 3 tablespoons / 27gr of grated parmesan cheese
- 3 cups / 550gr of spring mix greens
- 6 halved cherry tomatoes
- 2 medium egg yolks
- ¼ cup / 55gr of butter
- 1 teaspoon / 5ml of lemon juice
- 3 medium eggs, poached
- 1 tablespoon / 0.45gr of dried chives

## Directions

| | |
|---|---|
| **1.** | Cook bacon to desired crispiness, drain and cool. |
| **2.** | Lightly spray some non-stick spray onto a microwave safe plate. To the plate add the parmesan cheese in 3 separate mounds. Microwave until the mounds are crispy. Take out the microwave and allow to cool. |
| **3.** | Add the egg yolks and lemon juice to a blender and blend until the mixture is a pale yellow. |
| **4.** | Microwave the butter until it starts to bubble. Add this melted butter to the blender mixture and blend until combined. Should be light in color and thicken as it cools. |
| **5.** | Put the greens, tomatoes and bacon slices on to a plate. |
| **6.** | Add a layer of parmesan cheese on top. |
| **7.** | Add the poached eggs on top of the cheese and pour your hollandaise sauce over them. |
| **8.** | Garnish with chives. |

**Serves: 1** kCal: 434 | Carbs: 5.7g | Fat: 32.3g | Protein: 27.6g

## Ingredients

- 4oz / 115gr of halloumi cheese
- 2 teaspoons/ 9½gr of mayonnaise
- ¼ cup / 45gr of spinach
- 4 leaves of basil, torn
- 0.8oz / 23gr of sliced cucumber
- 6 whole blackberries, sliced in half

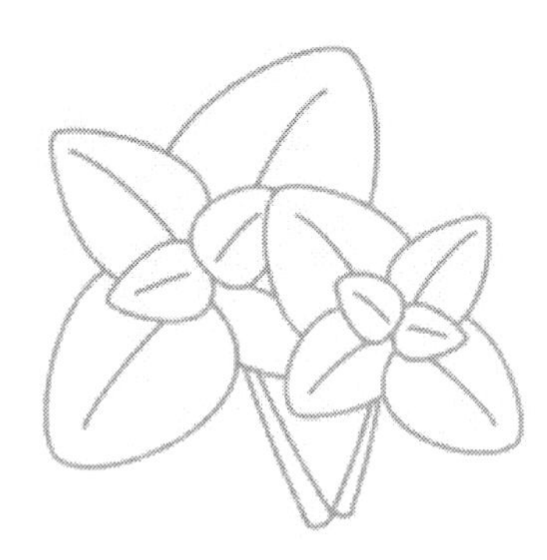

## Directions

| | |
|---|---|
| 1. | Warm up your Panini press to a medium heat. |
| 2. | Slice the halloumi into equal-sized rectangles. |
| 3. | Put the halloumi on the Panini press and cook until it starts to brown. |
| 4. | Flip the halloumi and brown the other sides. |
| 5. | On one of the halloumi slices, Layer the mayo, spinach, cucumber, basil, and blackberries. |
| 6. | Take the other halloumi slice and place it on top of the fillings to make a sandwich. |
| 7. | Close the press and hold for one minute. |
| 8. | Switch off the press. |
| 9. | Plate the halloumi sandwich, top with any remaining berries and serve warm. |

# DINNER

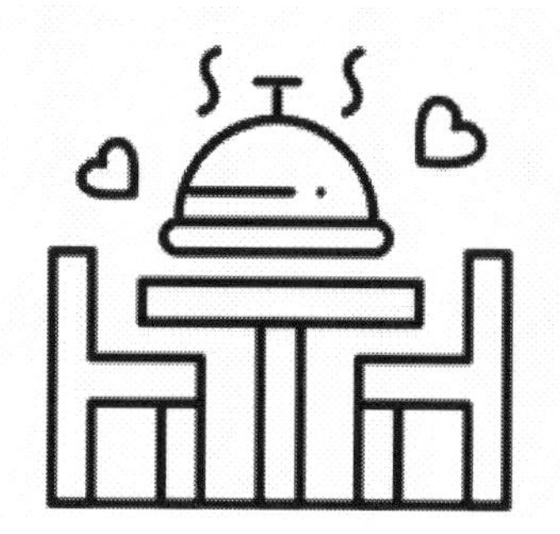

# IN-A-SKILLET PHILLY CHEESESTEAK

**Serves: 5** kCal: 535.74 | Carbs: 8.72g | Fat: .35.64g | Protein: 42.74g

## Ingredients

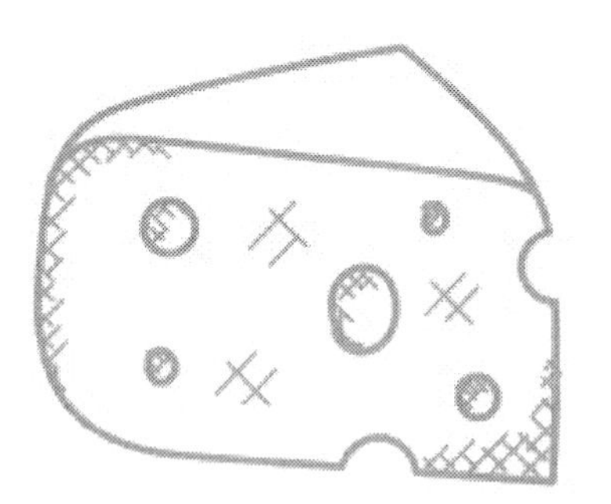

- 1 tablespoon / 15ml of olive oil
- 1 medium-sized onion, cut in half
- 2 teaspoons / 10gr of mince garlic
- 1 cup / 250gr of green bell-pepper, diced
- 1lb / 455gr of ground beef
- 1 teaspoon / 5gr of salt
- ¼ teaspoon / 2gr of black pepper
- ¼ teaspoon / 2gr of garlic powder
- ¼ teaspoon / 2gr of onion powder
- ½ cup / 120ml of beef broth
- 1b / 455gr of cauliflower florets
- 8oz / 227gr of sliced mushrooms
- ¼ cup of half and half
- 10 slices of provolone cheese

## Directions

| | |
|---|---|
| 1. | Dice one half of the onion and thinly slice the other half. |
| 2. | In a large skillet, add the olive oil. Once it's heated, add half of the onion, the garlic, and half of the bell-pepper. Sauté until the veggies begin to soften. |
| 3. | Add the ground beef and season it with the onion powder, garlic powder, salt and half of the black pepper. Crumble the beef with a potato masher. |
| 4. | Cover the skillet and cook for a few more mins, stirring now and then until the beef is completely cooked. |
| 5. | Add the beef broth, cauliflower, onions, bell-pepper and mushrooms and stir. Allow to simmer for 15 mins and then mash the cauliflower into smaller pieces. |
| 6. | Turn off the heat and stir in the half and half. |
| 7. | Season with the remaining pepper, onion and garlic powders. |
| 8. | Spread the cheese slices over the top and cover with a lid. |
| 9. | Cook until the cheese has melted. |

# INSTANT POT FAUX-LASAGNA

**Serves: 8** kCal: 403.24 | Carbs: 7.36g | Fat: 26.85g | Protein: 30.9g

## Ingredients

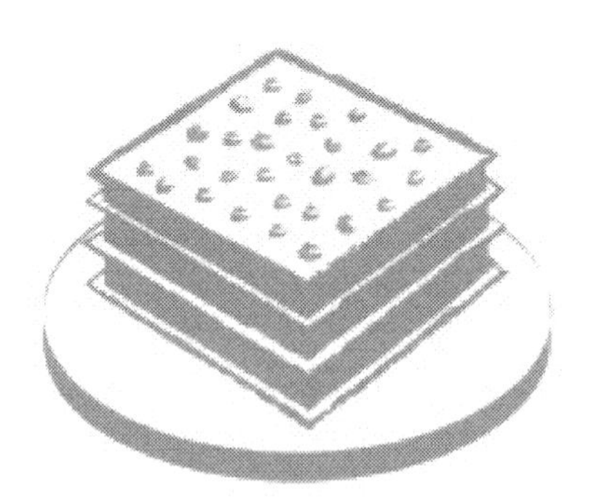

- 1lb / 450gr of ground beef
- 2 cloves of minced garlic
- 1small diced onion
- 1½ cup / 340gr of ricotta cheese
- ½ cup / 70gr of parmesan cheese
- 2 large eggs
- 25oz / 740ml of marinara sauce
- 8oz / 230gr of sliced mozzarella cheese
- 1 cup / 235ml of water

## Directions

| | |
|---|---|
| **1.** | Set your Instant Pot to the sauté setting and brown the beef, garlic and onion. |
| **2.** | In a mixing bowl, mix the ricotta, parmesan and eggs together well. |
| **3.** | Switch off the Instant Pot, remove the beef and drain the grease. |
| **4.** | Add the marinara to the beef and mix well. Leave some sauce for the top of the dish. |
| **5.** | Take out a spring-form pan and wrap the base with foil. The spring-form pan must be able to fit in to the Instant Pot. |
| **6.** | On the spring-form pan, layer your meat, mozzarella cheese and ricotta, until everything is in the pan. |
| **7.** | Top off with the left over marinara sauce. |
| **8.** | Over the pan loosely with some foil. |
| **9.** | Add the cup of water to the Instant Pot, then the rack and then the spring-form pan onto the rack. |
| **10.** | Close the Instant Pot lid and valve and cook on a high pressure for 9 minutes. |
| **11.** | Release the valve and serve. |

# CHICKEN SALAD WITH BACON

**Serves: 4** kCal: 725.12 | Carbs: 5.38g | Fat: 57.29g | Protein: 37.86g

## Ingredients

- 2 tablespoons / 24gr of olive oil
- 1.1oz / 500gr of chicken breast filets, cut into cubes
- 1 clove of minced garlic
- 5 slices of chopped bacon
- 1 cup / 65gr of sliced mushrooms
- □ cup / 43gr of fresh basil
- 5oz / 140gr of fresh spinach
- 3 – 4 small-sized sun-dried tomatoes
- 1 cup / 235ml of sugar-free ranch dressing

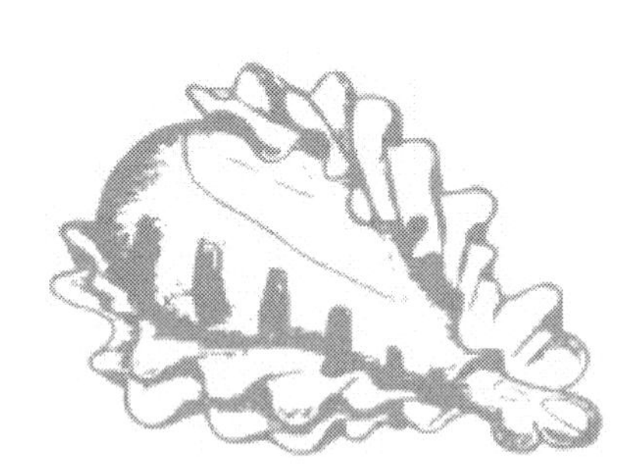

## Directions

| | |
|---|---|
| **1.** | Put a frying pan over a medium heat and add the olive oil. |
| **2.** | Once the oil is hot, add the chicken cubes and brown them. |
| **3.** | Just before the chicken is done, add the garlic and mix well. Cook until the chicken is done. |
| **4.** | Take the chicken out of the pan and put into a mixing bowl. Set aside. |
| **5.** | Add bacon to the same pan and cook until it's reached your desired crispiness. Once done, add to the chicken. |
| **6.** | Add the mushrooms, basil and some of the spinach to the chicken and bacon and mix until the spinach wilts. |
| **7.** | Put the remaining spinach into a serving bowl and spread the chicken mix over the top. |
| **8.** | Garnish with the tomatoes and ranch dressing. |

**Serves: 3**

kCal: 512.07 | Carbs: 6.77g | Fat: 35.83g | Protein: 37.23g

## Ingredients

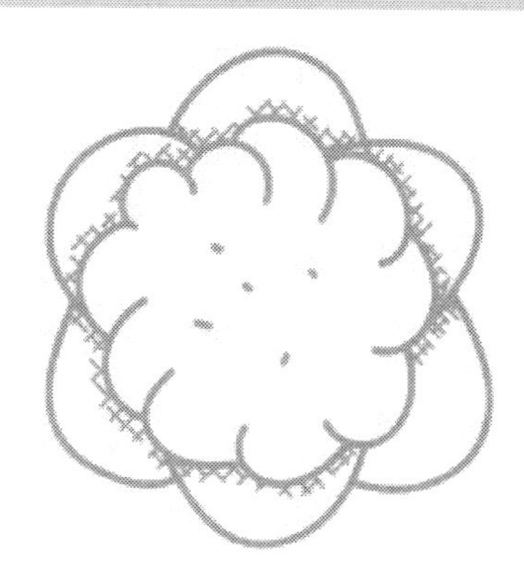

- 3 cups / 700gr of cauliflower florets
- 1 tablespoon / 15gr of butter
- 3 tablespoons / 45ml of almond milk (preferably unsweetened)
- 12oz / 340gr ground beef
- ¼ cup / 32gr of almond flour
- 2teaspoons / 2gr of chopped fresh parsley
- 2 teaspoons / 10ml of Worcestershire sauce
- ¼ teaspoon / 2gr of onion powder
- ¼ teaspoon / 2gr of garlic powder
- Salt and pepper for tasting
- 1 tablespoon / 15ml of olive oil
- 1½ cup / 100gr of sliced mushrooms
- ¼ cup / 60ml of beef broth
- 2 tablespoons / 15gr of sour cream

## Directions

| | |
|---|---|
| 1. | Preheat the oven to 375ºF / 190ºC and line a baking sheet with foil. |
| 2. | Boil a pot of water, liberally seasoning with salt. Add the cauliflower and boil until tender. |
| 3. | Drain the cauliflower and put it into a mixing bowl. Add the butter and almond milk and mash it up. |
| 4. | In a separate mixing bowl, mix the beef, flour, Worcester sauce, onion powder, garlic powder, salt, pepper and parsley together well. |
| 5. | Divide the beef mixture into burger patties shapes to create your "steaks" and place them on the lined baking sheet. Bake until the "steaks" are cooked through. |
| 6. | Place a large skillet over a medium-high heat and add the olive oil. |
| 7. | Add the mushrooms and cook until they are brown and tender. |
| 8. | Add the beef broth, stirring often, scraping the bits forming on the bottom. |
| 9. | Add the sour cream and whisk to combine. Season with some salt and pepper |
| 10. | Serve the "Salisbury Steaks" on top of the cauli mash and top it off with the mushroom sauce. |

**Serves: 3** kCal: 434.24 | Carbs: 5.47g | Fat: 41.01g | Protein: 10.03g

## Ingredients

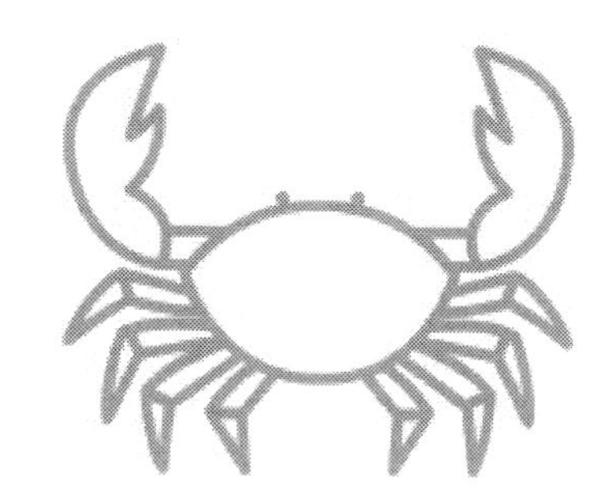

- 1 can of hearts of palm. Drain the liquid.
- 2 tablespoons / 30ml of mayonnaise
- 1 teaspoon / 5gr of Old Bay seasoning
- 1 tablespoon / 1gr of parsley
- ¼ cup / 32gr of almond flour
- 1 large beaten egg
- 1 tablespoon / 10gr of diced onion
- 1 teaspoon / 5gr of butter
- 3 tablespoons / 42gr of almond meal
- 2 tablespoons / 18gr of parmesan cheese
- 4 tablespoons / 60ml of avocado oil

## Directions

| | |
|---|---|
| **1.** | Shred the hearts of palm with a fork, until it resembles crab meat. |
| **2.** | Add the Old Bay seasoning, mayo, almond flour, egg and parsley and mix until combined. |
| **3.** | Heat the butter over a medium heat in a skillet, and sauté the diced onion until it's translucent. Gently fold the onions into the hearts of palm "crab meat". |
| **4.** | In a shallow bowl, mix together the almond meal and parmesan for a coating. |
| **5.** | Separate the "crab meat" into 6 equal balls and press into the coating, squashing the balls into cakes. Make sure the cakes are completely covered. |
| **6.** | Heat a skillet over a medium-high heat and add the avocado oil. |
| **7.** | Fry each cake, turning carefully to brown each side. Preferably fry two at a time. |
| **8.** | Serve hot. |

**Serves: 2** kCal: 328.8 | Carbs: 5.45g | Fat: 29.95g | Protein: 5.45g

## Ingredients

### For the Marinade

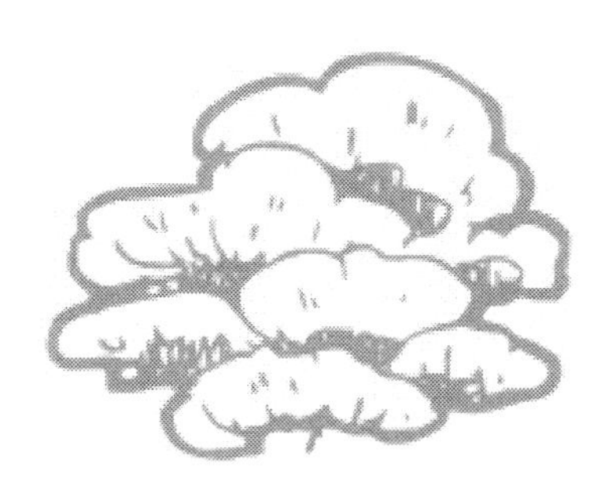

- 2 tablespoons / 30ml of avocado oil
- 1 tablespoon / 15ml of liquid aminos
- 1 teaspoon / 5ml of liquid smoke
- 2 cloves of minced garlic
- ½ teaspoon / 5gr of cumin
- 1 teaspoon / 5ml of balsamic vinegar

### For the Mushrooms

- 2 large Portobello mushroom caps
- 1 medium-sized diced avocado
- ½ of a medium-sized roma tomato, diced
- ½ cup / 20gr of finely minced parlsey
- 2 tablespoons / 28gr of hulled hemp seeds
- ½ teaspoon / 2.5gr of salt

## Directions

| | |
|---|---|
| 1. | In a small mixing bowl, whisk all the marinade Ingredients together. |
| 2. | Clean and trim the mushrooms, including the stem if desired. |
| 3. | Using a shallow dish, soak the mushrooms with the marinade and ensure they are completely coated. Let them rest in the marinade, turning occasionally, for about 5 minutes. |
| 4. | In a separate mixing bowl, combine the avocado, tomato and parsley. Sprinkle some salt and half of the hemp seeds over this. Toss to evenly coat. |
| 5. | Preheat a skillet over a medium-high heat and pan sear the mushrooms, until each side is browed and the mushrooms are tender. |
| 6. | Top each mushroom with the avo salsa and residual hemp seeds and serve. |

**Serves: 5**

kCal: 420.82 | Carbs: 7.12g | Fat: 36.7g | Protein: 16.42g

## Ingredients

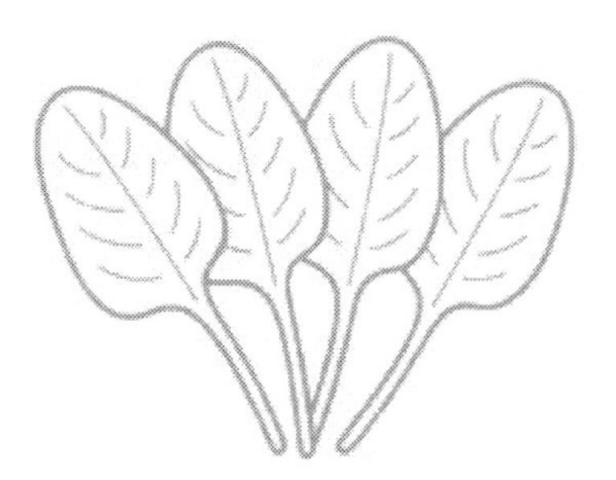

- 2 medium-sized zucchini
- 1½ cups / 375gr of ricotta
- 1 cup / 235gr of parmesan cheese. Divide in half.
- 2 teaspoons / 1gr of dried basil
- 1medium-sized egg
- 4 tablespoons / 57gr of butter
- 2 medium-sized cloves of garlic, minced
- 1 cup / 950ml heavy cream
- ½ cup / 30gr baby spinach, chopped roughly
- ½ oz / 7gr of sun-dried tomatoes

## Directions

| | |
|---|---|
| 1. | Preheat your oven to 350ºF / 180ºC. |
| 2. | Spray non-stick spray over a casserole dish. |
| 3. | Slice each zucchini lengthwise with a wide vegetable peeler to make "ribbons". You will need about 20 "ribbons" to fill a small casserole dish. |
| 4. | In a large mixing bowl, add the ricotta, half of the parmesan, basil, spinach and egg and mix well. Place in a large freezer bag and set aside for later. This bag will be used as a piping bag, so make sure it's adequate. (Use a piping bag if you have one) |
| 5. | In a saucepan, heat the butter, garlic and cream over a medium heat. Add the remaining parmesan and stir until the sauce has thickened. Take off from the heat. |
| 6. | Pour a third of the sauce into the bottom of the casserole dish. |
| 7. | Secure the top of the freezer bag / piping bag and cut the tip as if you're going to pipe some frosting. Squeeze / pipe the mixture over the zucchini "ribbons". |
| 8. | Roll each strip gently, so as not to squeeze the filling out. |
| 9. | Place each zucchini curl sideways into the sauce in the casserole dish. |
| 10. | Add the sundried tomatoes to the remaining sauce and stir. |
| 11. | Pour the sauce over the zucchini curl. |
| 12. | Cover the dish with some foil and bake for 25 – 30 mins until the top of the sauce is browned and bubbling. |
| 13. | Take out the oven, allow to cool slightly and serve. |

# CHICKEN MEATLOAF CUPCAKES

**Serves: 6**

kCal: 316.568 | Carbs: 2.72g | Fat: 23.87g | Protein: 24.82g

## Ingredients

### Buffalo Gravy

- 1½ tablespoons / 21gr of unsalted butter
- 1 medium-sized minced garlic clove
- □ cup / 150gr of wing sauce
- 1 teaspoon / 5ml of Worcestershire sauce
- 1½ tablespoons / 22ml of white vinegar
- Salt and pepper for tasting

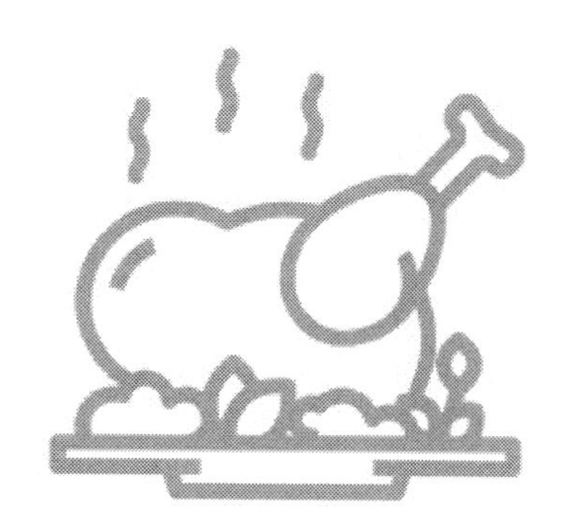

### For the Chicken

- 1 tablespoon / 15ml of extra-virgin olive oil
- ½ a medium-sized diced onion
- ½ cup / 50gr of minced celery
- 1lb / 455gr of ground chicken
- 1 teaspoon / 5ml of Worcester sauce
- 2 medium-sized minced garlic cloves
- ½ cup / 110gr of crushed pork rinds
- Salt and pepper for tasting
- 1 large egg
- 2 tablespoons / 30ml of chicken broth
- ½ teaspoon / 2.3gr of unflavored gelatin
- ¼ teaspoon / 0.54gr of celery seed
- 2oz / 55gr blue cheese
- 2½ tablespoons / 36gr of unsalted butter

## Directions

| | |
|---|---|
| **1.** | Preheat your oven to 375ºF / 190ºC. |
| **2.** | Over a low heat, melt the gravy butter in a saucepan. |
| **3.** | Add the 1 garlic and cook for a minute. Add the wing sauce, Worcestershire sauce, vinegar, salt and pepper to the garlic and whisk to combine. Simmer for a minute and set aside. |
| **4.** | In a skillet over a medium heat, warm the olive oil, add the onion, celery and 2 garlic. Cook until soft and set aside to cool down. |
| **5.** | In a mixing bowl, whisk the egg and chicken broth together. Add the gelatin and allow to bloom for 5 mins. |
| **6.** | In the bowl with the onion mixture, add the chicken, Worcestershire sauce, celery seed, pork rinds, salt, pepper and a quarter of the prepared wing sauce. Add the whisked egg and mix to combine. |
| **7.** | Spray a cupcake tin with some non-stick spray and add about 2 tablespoons of the mixture to each cupcake spot. Using your finger, make a space in the center of each one and add blue cheese and a slice of butter. Top each one with the remaining meat mixture and brush some wing sauce over the lid. |
| **8.** | Put it in the oven and bake for 25 minutes, brushing more sauce on top every 10 minutes. |

Serves: 4 kCal: 315.05 | Carbs: 5.89g | Fat: 25.23g | Protein: 17.43g

## Ingredients

### For the Caulirice

- 1 teaspoon / 5gr of coconut oil
- ½ cup / 110gr of coconut flakes, unsweetened
- 2 cups / 480gr of cauliflower florets

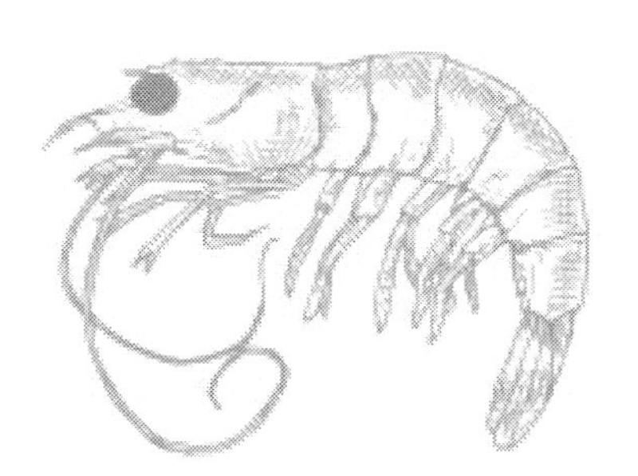

### For the Shrimp

- 1 teaspoon / 5gr of coconut oil
- ¼ of a medium-sized diced sweet onion
- 2 medium-sized minced garlic cloves
- 1¼ cups / 300ml of canned coconut milk
- 24 medium-sized tail on precooked shrimp, frozen
- 3 sprigs of chopped cilantro
- ½ of a medium-sized lime, juiced
- 2 tablespoons / 28gr of crushed red pepper

## Directions

| | |
|---|---|
| **1.** | Warm up a non-stick skillet for the caulirice. |
| **2.** | Heat the coconut oil and sauté the coconut flakes until slightly brown. |
| **3.** | Add the cauliflower florets to a food processer / blender and pulse until it looks like rice. |
| **4.** | Add the caulirice to the skillet and stir. |
| **5.** | Sauté until the coconut is toasted and the caulirice is softened |
| **6.** | Don't be tempted to add extra liquid, just let it fry in the coconut oil. |
| **7.** | Take the caulirice and coconut out of the skillet and place in a covered container until ready for serving. |
| **8.** | In the same skillet, add the coconut oil, garlic and onion and sauté until aromatic. |
| **9.** | Add in the coconut milk and stir until it simmers |
| **10.** | Allow it to reduce for 5 mins. |
| **11.** | Add the shrimp to the coconut sauce and cook on a medium-low heat until the shrimp is tender and begins to curl. |
| **12.** | Add the lime juice and cilantro and gently stir. |
| **13.** | Dust the red pepper over the shrimp. |
| **14.** | Dish up the caulirice, layer the shrimp on top and drizzle with sauce. |

# COCONUT AVOCADO SMOOTHIE

**Serves: 4** kCal: 252.75 | Carbs: 3.7g | Fat: 26.25g | Protein: 2.68g

## Ingredients

- 1 medium-sized avocado, cut in half
- 14oz / 400gr can of coconut milk
- 2½ tablespoons / 25gr of allulose
- 2oz / 60ml of water
- 8oz / 227gr of ice cubes
- ¼ tablespoon / 5½gr of vanilla bean extract

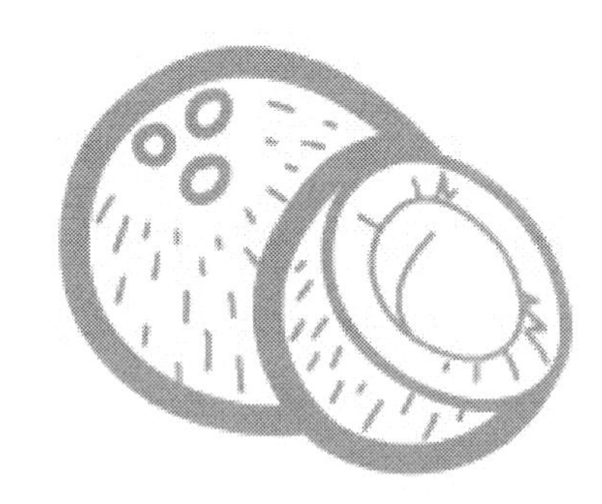

## Directions

| | |
|---|---|
| **1.** | If you notice that the coconut milk has separate, just whisk together until it's fully incorporated. |
| **2.** | Using a blender or a smoothie maker, add the avocado halves, coconut milk, allulose, water, ice and vanilla. |
| **3.** | Blend until thick and smooth. |
| **4.** | Pour into a glass and serve. You can top it off with some whipped coconut cream or grilled coconut cubes to make it more decadent. |
| **5.** | This smoothie is a great option for fat boosting your keto diet |

Serves: 3 kCal: 187.07 | Carbs: 4.53g | Fat: 11.47g | Protein: 6.27g

## Ingredients

- ½ cup / 81gr of chia seeds
- 1½ cups / 355ml of unsweetened almond milk
- 2 tablespoons / 28gr of monk fruit sweetener
- 1 teaspoon / 5ml of vanilla extract
- 4 medium-sized diced strawberries
- 2 teaspoons / 10gr of unsweetened cocoa powder

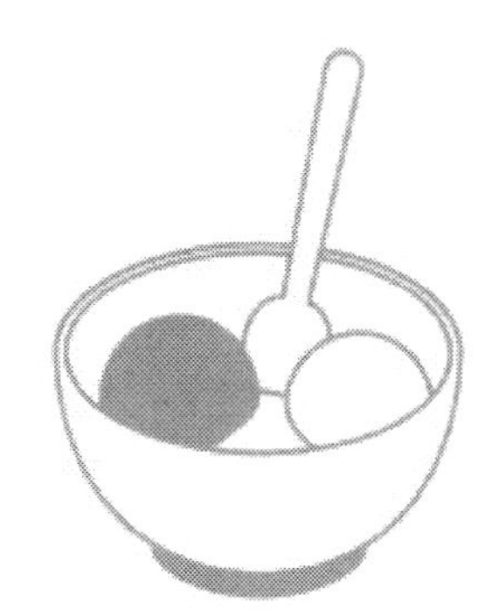

## Directions

| | |
|---|---|
| 1. | In a mixing bowl, mix the chia seeds, almond milk, sweetener and vanilla together. Leave to chill in the fridge for 10 – 15 mins until firm. |
| 2. | Take out the fridge and divide equally between three bowls. |
| 3. | To one of the bowls, add the cocoa powder and mix. Taste and add more sweetener if required. |
| 4. | Cook the strawberries in the microwave for 30 seconds until soft and mash with a fork. |
| 5. | Mix the mashed strawberries into another chia seed bowl. |
| 6. | You will now have one bowl of chocolate, one bowl of strawberry and one bowl of vanilla, which will form your layers. |
| 7. | In small glasses, layer each one repeatedly. You can even lay some sliced strawberries against the sides of the glass, as you layer up. |

**Serves: 12** kCal: 58.92 | Carbs: 0.83g | Fat: 5.01g | Protein: 2.31g

## Ingredients

- 2 large egg whites
- 8 tablespoons / 114gr of allulose
- 1 cup / 70gr of sliced almonds
- ¼ cup / 55gr of unsweetened coconut flakes

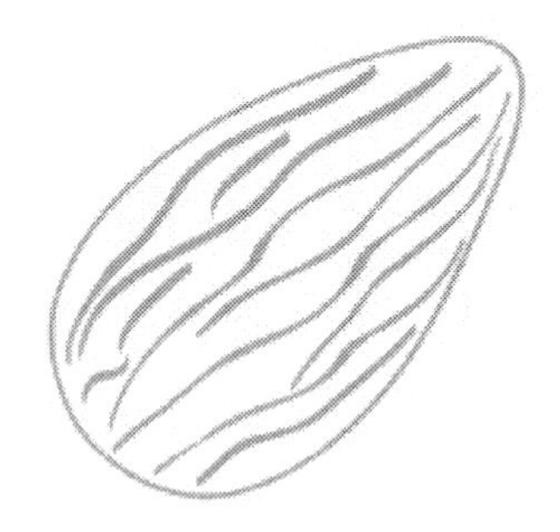

## Directions

| | |
|---|---|
| **1.** | Set your oven to 325ºF / 162ºC |
| **2.** | Line some baking sheets with baking paper. |
| **3.** | In a mixing bowl, combine the egg whites and the allulose. |
| **4.** | Add the sweetener and whisk until the mixture thick. Must not be foamy. |
| **5.** | Add the sliced almonds and coconut flakes and stir until combined. |
| **6.** | Whip mixture until it resembles a cookie batter. |
| **7.** | Scoop the batter into mound and place on the lined baking sheet, spacing the mounds evenly. |
| **8.** | Flatten the mounds to form cookies. |
| **9.** | Bake for 10 mins and turn the baking sheet around to get an even bake. |
| **10.** | Bake for a further 8 mins until the cookies are toasted and crispy. |
| **11.** | Take out and leave to cool. |

Serves: 8

kCal: 222.38 | Carbs: 6.88g | Fat: 21.09g | Protein: 2.07g

## Ingredients

- 1 medium-sized avocado
- 1 can of coconut milk
- ½ cup / 120ml of heavy cream
- ¾ cup / 96gr of allulose
- 1 medium-sized lime
- 1 cup / 220gr of coconut flakes

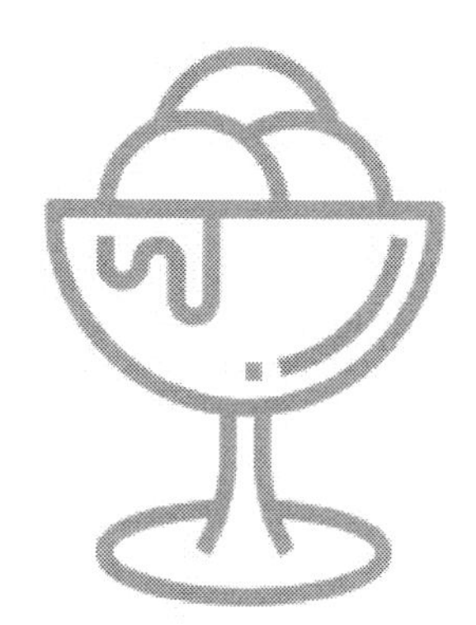

## Directions

| | |
|---|---|
| 1. | Cut the avo, remove the stone and scoop out the avo insides. Add it to a blender. |
| 2. | Along with the avo, add the coconut milk, cream, and allulose and blend until smooth. |
| 3. | Take the line and juice and zest it. Add the juice and zest to the blender and blend again for a minute. |
| 4. | Place in the fridge for a minimum of an hour. |
| 5. | Add the coconut flakes to a warm pan and toast until lightly brown around the edges. Take off the heat. |
| 6. | Take out your ice cream machine and add the chilled avo mixture to it. Churn according to the machines' Directions. |
| 7. | Place it in a freezer safe container and freeze. |
| 8. | When ready to serve, garnish with some coconut flakes. |

# COCOCHOC MUG CAKE

**Serves: 2** kCal: 219 | Carbs: 2.95g | Fat: 19.06g | Protein: 7.23g

## Ingredients

- 2 tablespoons / 14gr of coconut flour
- 2 tablespoons / 15gr of cocoa powder
- 2 tablespoons / 15gr of Swerve confectioners (or erythritol)
- ¼ teaspoon / 2gr of baking powder
- 2 large eggs
- 2 tablespoons / 30gr of melted butter
- 2 tablespoons / 30ml of unsweetened almond milk

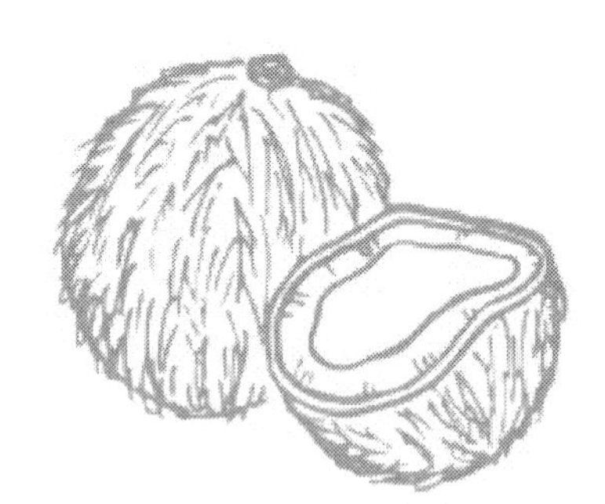

## Directions

| | |
|---|---|
| **1.** | Mix together the coconut flour, cocoa powder, sweetener and baking powder. |
| **2.** | Add the eggs, butter, and almond milk and mix well. |
| **3.** | Grease a large coffee mug and pour in the cake batter. |
| **4.** | Place in the center of your microwave and cook for 2 minutes. Keep an eye, as every microwave is different. When you see the cake popping over the top of the mug, it's done. |
| **5.** | Carefully take out of the microwave as it can be hot. |
| **6.** | Remove from the mug, slice in half and serve. |

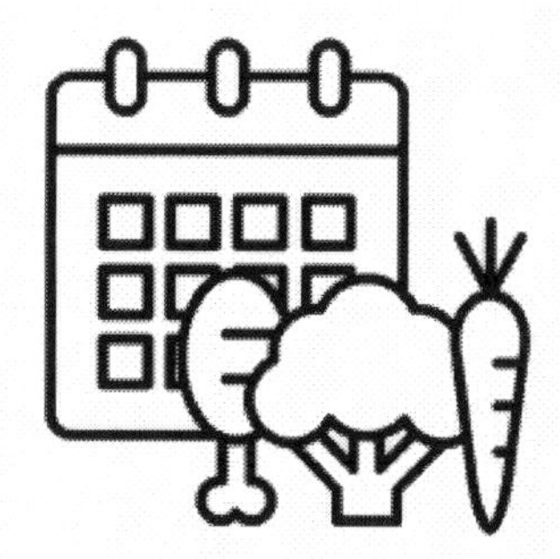

*indicates a new meal not mentioned previously in this book

## Breakfast*: Coconut and Berry Oatmeal

Calories: 445 | Carbohydrates: 6.34g | Fat: 38.16g | Protein: 10.45g

## Ingredients

- 2 tablespoons / 28gr of ground flaxseed
- 1 tablespoon / 14gr of almond meal
- 1 tablespoon / 14gr of desiccated coconut
- ½ teaspoon / 2½gr of vanilla powder
- ½ teaspoon / 2½gr of cinnamon
- □ cup / 80ml of coconut milk
- ½ cup / 120ml of almond milk
- ¼ cup / 85gr of mixed berries
- 1 teaspoon / 5gr of dried pumpkin seeds

## Directions

| | |
|---|---|
| **1.** | Place a saucepan on the stove to preheat it. |
| **2.** | Add everything except the berries and pumpkin seeds to the saucepan. |
| **3.** | Stir continuously until the mixture is hot and thick like oatmeal |
| **4.** | Pour the mixture into a bowl, add the berries and seeds and serve. |

***Lunch: Steak and Mushroom Stroganoff***

***Dinner: Chicken Salad with Bacon***

*Breakfast: Breakfast Bowl*

## Lunch*: Casserole Sub Sandwich

Calories: 312.43 | Carbohydrates:3.12 g | Fat: 22.11g | Protein: 24.91g

## Ingredients

- 8oz / 227gr of smoked deli ham slices
- 8 slices of swiss cheese
- 16 slices of dill pickles
- 3 tablespoons / 45ml of Italian dressing
- ¼ tablespoon / 7½ ml of Italian seasoning

## Directions

| | |
|---|---|
| 1. | Preheat the oven to 375ºF / 190ºC |
| 2. | In a casserole dish, spread out the ham slices in a layer. |
| 3. | Add a layer of swiss cheese on top of the ham. |
| 4. | Add the dill pickles, dressing and seasoning. |
| 5. | Bake for 10 – 15 minutes until the cheese has melted |

*Dinner: Faux Crab Cakes*

*Breakfast: Blueberry Pancake Bites*

*Lunch: Bacon Salad with Kale*

## Dinner*: Cheese and Broccoli Soup

Calories: 418.85 | Carbohydrates: 5.62g Fat | 38.68g | Protein: 12.45g

## Ingredients

- 1 tablespoon / 15gr of butter
- 1 small-sized onion, chopped
- 2medium-sized cloves of garlic, minced
- Salt and pepper for tasting
- ½ teaspoon / 2½gr of xanthan gum
- ½ cup / 120ml of chicken broth
- 1 cup / 184gr of broccoli, chopped
- 1 cup / 240ml of heavy cream
- 1½ cup / 180gr of grated cheddar cheese

## Directions

| | |
|---|---|
| 1. | Preheat a pot on a medium heat. |
| 2. | Add the butter, onions, garlic, salt and pepper to the pot and sauté until the onions are see-through |
| 3. | Sprinkle the xanthan gum over the onions mixture. |
| 4. | Pour in the chicken broth and stir. |
| 5. | Add the broccoli to the pot and make sure the broth coats all the veg. |
| 6. | Add the cream and stir quickly and frequently, ensuring the xanthan gum gets mixed in and thickens. Bring to a boil. |
| 7. | Add the cheese and slowly whisk until all has melted. |
| 8. | Dish into soup bowls, garnish with broccoli and cheese and serve. |

## Breakfast*: Cheese and Mushroom Omelette

Calories: 515 | Carbohydrates: 4.17 g | Fat: 39.58g | Protein: 21.34g

## Ingredients

- 3 large eggs
- 2 teaspoons / 10ml of heavy cream
- 3oz/ 85gr of mushrooms, sliced
- 1 teaspoon / 5ml of olive oil
- 2oz / 56gr of crumbled goats cheese
- Some Spike seasoning for taste
- Optional green onions for garnishing

## Directions

| | |
|---|---|
| **1.** | Heat the oil in a frying pan and fry the mushrooms until soft. |
| **2.** | Whisk together the eggs, heavy cream and some Spike seasoning. |
| **3.** | Remove the mushrooms from the pan and set aside. |
| **4.** | Add the egg mixture to the pan and cook for 2 to 3 minutes. |
| **5.** | When you see the egg starting to set, add the cooked mushrooms and goats cheese. |
| **6.** | Carefully fold the omelette over and cook until the goats cheese begins melting. |
| **7.** | Serve and garnish with green onions, if desired. |

***Lunch:* *Bacon Cheeseburger Kebabs***

***Dinner:* *Salisbury Steak and Cauli Mash***

*Breakfast: Spicy Eggs and Cheesy Hash*

## Lunch*: Avo Bowls

Calories: 169.13 | Carbohydrates: 2.53g | Fat: 14.52g | Protein: 3.27g

### Ingredients

- 3 medium-sized avocados, chopped in half, stones removed
- 1½oz / 50gr of chopped mushrooms
- 1 medium-sized chopped green onion
- 10 chopped cherry tomatoes
- 1oz / 44gr of crumbled goats cheese
- 1 tablespoon / 15ml of olive oil
- 1 tablespoon / 15ml of liquid smoke
- ½ teaspoon / 2½gr of paprika
- 3 tablespoons / 45ml of balsamic vinegar

### Directions

| | |
|---|---|
| 1. | Place a frying pan over a medium heat to warm. |
| 2. | In a mixing bowl, add the mushrooms, onions and tomatoes. |
| 3. | In the warmed pan, heat the olive oil, liquid smoke and paprika. |
| 4. | Add the goats cheese to the pan, and sauté until the cheese has browned. |
| 5. | Take the pan off the stove and add the goats cheese to the mixing bowl. Mix together. |
| 6. | Scoop out a portion of the avo halves to make room for the filling. |
| 7. | Spoon the mixture into the holes in the avos. Garnish with the scooped portion of avo. |
| 8. | Pour a ½ teaspoon of balsamic vinegar onto each and serve. |

*Dinner: Shrimp and Caulirice*

*Breakfast: Chorizo Baked Eggs*

*Lunch: Steak and Mushroom Stroganoff*

## Dinner*: Creamy Chicken

Calories: 382.79 | Carbohydrates: 4.33g | Fat: 25.93g | Protein: 31.85g

## Ingredients

- 2 slices of chopped bacon
- 2lb / 910gr of chicken breast filets (boneless and skinless)
- 16oz / 450gr of cream cheese
- ½ cup / 120ml of water
- 2 tablespoons/ 30ml of apple cider vinegar
- 1 tablespoon / 0.45gr of dried chives
- 1½ teaspoon / 5gr onion powder
- 1½ teaspoon / 5gr garlic powder
- 1 teaspoon / 2½gr of crushed red pepper flakes
- 1 teaspoon / 2½gr of dried dill
- Salt and pepper for tasting
- 2oz / 55gr of grated cheddar cheese
- 1 medium-sized sliced green onion

## Directions

| | |
|---|---|
| **1.** | Set your Instant Pot to the sauté and allow to heat up. Add the bacon and cook until its crisp. Take the bacon out and set aside, hitting cancel on your Instant Pot. |
| **2.** | Add the chicken, cream cheese, water, vinegar, chives, garlic powder, onion powder, red pepper flakes, dill, salt and pepper to the Instant Pot. |
| **3.** | Manually set it to high pressure for 15 minutes. Once done, do a quick release. |
| **4.** | Remove the chicken and shred it. When done, return it to the pot. |
| **5.** | Add in the cheddar and stir. |
| **6.** | Dish up the mixture, sprinkle the bacon and green onions on top and serve. |

*Breakfast: Breakfast Bowl*

## Lunch*: Taco Salad

Calories: 388.37 | Carbohydrates: 6.5g | Fat: 32.47g | Protein: 15.8g

## Ingredients

- ¾lb / 340gr of ground beef
- 1 teaspoon / 5gr of ground cumin
- ½ teaspoon / 1.3gr of chili powder
- 1 teaspoon / ½gr of dried parsley
- 1teaspoon / 3gr of garlic powder
- 8oz / 227gr of chopped romaine lettuce
- 9oz / 255gr of chopped iceberg lettuce
- 2 small chopped red tomatoes
- 1½ cups / 180gr of grated mozzarella cheese
- 1 medium-sized chopped avocado
- 1 cup / 120gr of sour cream

## Directions

| | |
|---|---|
| 1. | Place the ground beef into a non-stick pan. |
| 2. | Add the herbs and spices to the beef and cook on a medium heat. |
| 3. | Once done, take off the heat and allow the beef to drain and cool. Set aside for later. |
| 4. | In a salad bowl, add the chopped lettuce, tomatoes, mozzarella and avocado and mix well. |
| 5. | Add the ground beef and sour cream on top of the salad mix and serve. |

*Dinner: Mushroom Steaks with Avo Salsa*

*Breakfast: Eggs Benedict Casserole*

*Lunch: Salmon Burgers on Cedar Plank*

## Dinner*: Chicken Cordon Bleu Soup

Calories: 580.17 | Carbohydrates: 3.93g | Fat: 50.74g | Protein: 27.43g

## Ingredients

- 6 small bacon strips
- 2 cups / 470ml of heavy whipping cream
- 6oz / 170gr of cream cheese
- 1 tablespoon / 14gr of butter
- 2 cups / 470ml of chicken stock
- 2 cups/ 200gr of grated Swiss cheese
- 1 cup / 150gr of ham, cubed
- 6oz / 170gr of chicken breast, shredded
- 2 cups / 134gr of chopped kale with stems removed

## Directions

| | |
|---|---|
| 1. | Over a medium-low heat, fry the bacon until crispy. Roughly chop it and set aside. Reserve about ¼ of the bacon for the garnish. |
| 2. | To a large soup pot, add the heavy cream, butter and cream cheese and heat over a medium heat. Cook until everything has melted. |
| 3. | Add the chicken stock to the soup pot and bring to a simmer. |
| 4. | Add the grated cheese and stir until completely melted. |
| 5. | Add the ham, chicken and ¾ of the bacon, mix and simmer. |
| 6. | Add the kale, stir and cook without the lid for 10mins, until the kale begins to soften. |
| 7. | Garnish with the bacon and serve hot. |

## Breakfast*: Breakfast Egg Wraps

Calories: 412 | Carbohydrates: 2.26 | Fat: 31.66 | Protein:28.21

## Ingredients

- 10 large eggs
- Salt
- Pepper
- 1½ cups / 510gr of grated cheddar
- 5 slices of cooked bacon
- 5 patties of cooked breakfast sausage

## Directions

| | |
|---|---|
| **1.** | Preheat a non-stick skillet on a medium-high heat. |
| **2.** | Take 2 of the eggs and whisk. |
| **3.** | Lower the heat to a medium-low, once the skillet is hot and add the whisked eggs. |
| **4.** | Greaseproof a muffin tin extremely well, as the mixture is very sticky. |
| **5.** | Season with some salt and pepper. |
| **6.** | Cover the skillet with a lid and allow the egg to cook almost all the way through. |
| **7.** | Sprinkle some cheese over the egg. |
| **8.** | Add a strip of bacon and half of a sausage patty on the egg. |
| **9.** | Carefully roll the egg over the fillings like a wrap. Take it slow, as it can be tricky. |
| **10.** | Set aside. |
| **11.** | Repeat all the steps for the next 4 egg wraps and serve. |

***Lunch: Tuna and Pesto Salad***

***Dinner: In-A-Skillet Philly Cheesesteak***

*Breakfast: Stuffed Peppers*

## Lunch*: Zucchini Salad

Calories: 206.4 | Carbohydrates: 4.33g | Fat: 14.59g | Protein: 11.55g

## Ingredients

- 2 medium-sized zucchinis
- 8 slices of cooked bacon
- 1 cup / 200gr of feta cheese, cubed
- 1 cup / 200gr of chopped cherry tomatoes
- 4 tablespoons / 60ml of balsamic vinegar

## Directions

| | |
|---|---|
| 1. | Slice the zucchinis into ribbons using a grater or a peeler. |
| 2. | In a salad bowl, add the zucchini ribbons and top off with the tomatoes, bacon and cheese. |
| 3. | Drizzle with the vinegar and toss before serving. |

*Dinner: Faux Crab Cakes*

*Breakfast: Ricotta and Blueberry Pancakes*

*Lunch: Cheesy Beer Soup*

## Dinner*: Cauli Casserole

Calories: 537.53 | Carbohydrates: 8.21g | Fat: 42.73g | Protein: 31.12g

## Ingredients

- 1 small-sized cauliflower
- 1 cup / 230gr of cream cheese
- 1 cup / 230gr of grated cheddar cheese
- 4 sliced of chopped bacon
- ¼ cup / 100gr of chopped mushrooms
- 1 medium-sized chopped jalapeno
- 2 medium-sized boneless, skinless, chicken thighs

## Directions

| | |
|---|---|
| 1. | Preheat your oven to 350ºF / 180ºC. |
| 2. | Chop the cauliflower into florets and add to a casserole dish. |
| 3. | In a mixing bowl, add the cream cheese, cheddar, jalapeno, mushrooms and bacon and mix well. |
| 4. | Add the cheese mixture to the cauliflower and mix well. |
| 5. | Lay the chicken on the cauliflower mixture and mix gently. |
| 6. | Bake for one hour, until the cheese has melted and the chicken has cooked. |

## Breakfast*: Pizza Eggs

Calories: 333 | Carbohydrates: 4.28g | Fat: 22.66g | Protein: 25.59g

## Ingredients

- 3 large eggs, separated
- 4 tablespoons / 57gr of grated mozzarella cheese
- 1 teaspoon / 5gr of Italian herb blend
- 2 large sliced black olives
- 4 large mild pepper rings
- 1 tablespoon / 15gr of diced red bell-pepper
- 1 tablespoon / 15gr of tomato sauce (preferably Rao's)

## Directions

| | |
|---|---|
| 1. | You will need 2 microwave-safe ramekin-sized bowls |
| 2. | Add 1 tablespoon of the mozzarella cheese and Italian herb seasoning to each bowl. |
| 3. | In a mixing bowl, beat the egg whites until just frothy, and pour into the bowls. |
| 4. | Microwave for 1-2 minutes until the whites are cooked. Allow to cool. |
| 5. | Beat the egg yolks and scramble lightly in a frying pan. |
| 6. | Fold the pizza toppings into the scrambled egg yolks and take off the heat. |
| 7. | Add some tomato sauce to your cooked egg white "pizza bases". |
| 8. | Add the scrambled egg mixture and remaining cheese on top of the tomato sauce. |
| 9. | Cook for another 20 seconds in the microwave, until the cheese has melted. |
| 10. | Serve hot. |

***Lunch: Taco-Stuffed Avos***

***Dinner: Chicken Salad with Bacon***

*Breakfast: Bacon Bagels*

## Lunch*: Vegan Scrambled No-Eggs

Calories: 211.4 | Carbohydrates: 4.74g | Fat: 17.56g | Protein: 10.09g

## Ingredients

- 14oz / 400gr of firm tofu
- 2 tablespoons / 28gr of diced yellow onion
- 3 tablespoons / 45ml of avocado oil
- 1½ tablespoons / 22½gr of nutritional yeast
- ½ teaspoon / 2½gr of garlic powder
- ½ teaspoon / 2½gr of turmeric
- ½ teaspoon / 2½gr of salt
- 1 cup / 340gr of baby spinach
- 3 diced grape tomatoes
- 3oz / 85gr of vegan cheddar

## Directions

| | |
|---|---|
| **1.** | You need to gently squeeze out some of the water in the tofu, so wrap it in some paper towels or a clean cloth and squeeze. |
| **2.** | On a medium heat, place a skillet and sauté the onion and a third of the avo oil, until the onion is soft. |
| **3.** | Add the tofu to the skillet and using a potato masher or a fork, crumble the tofu, until it resembles scrambled egg. |
| **4.** | Drizzle the remaining avo oil over the tofu. |
| **5.** | Sprinkle the tofu with the dry seasoning and stir to coat evenly. |
| **6.** | Cook over a medium heat, stirring and folding until most of the liquid has gone. |
| **7.** | Fold in the spinach, tomato and cheese and cook until the cheese has melted and the spinach has wilted. |
| **8.** | Serve hot. |
| **9.** | Leftovers can be stored in your fridge for 3 days. |

***Dinner: Chicken Meatloaf Cupcakes***

*Breakfast: Chicken and Waffle Sandwiches*

*Lunch: Pressed Halloumi with Blackberry, Basil and Spinach*

## Dinner*: Roast Chicken in Red pepper Gravy

Calories: 156 | Carbohydrates: 0% (1.2g) | Fat: 15% (10g) | Protein: 24% (12g)

## Ingredients

### Chicken Thighs

- 1½lb / 680gr of chicken thighs, boneless and skinless
- Salt and pepper for tasting
- 1 tablespoon / 15gr of coconut oil
- 4oz / 113gr of goats cheese
- 2 tablespoons / 5gr of chopped fresh parsley

### Roasted Red Pepper Gravy

- 4oz / 113gr of roasted red peppers
- 2 garlic cloves
- 2 tablespoons / 30ml of olive oil
- ½ cup / 120ml of heavy cream

## Directions

| | |
|---|---|
| 1. | Warm up your oven to 350°F / 180°C and place a skillet on a medium-high heat. |
| 2. | Season the chicken with salt and pepper. |
| 3. | Put the coconut oil in the skillet to melt. Once melted, add the chicken and sear for 5 mins on each side, until browned. |
| 4. | Add the red peppers, garlic and olive oil to a blender and puree everything. Add the heavy cream and blend again until thoroughly combined. |
| 5. | Take the skillet off the heat and pour the gravy over the chicken. Flip the chicken and coat evenly in the gravy. |
| 6. | Sprinkle the goats cheese over the chicken. |
| 7. | Place the skillet in the oven to bake the chicken for 10-15 minutes. |
| 8. | Garnish with some fresh parsley and serve. |

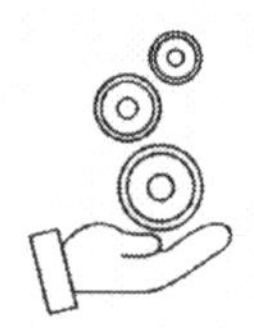

1. **Set realistic goals for yourself:** Reading stories of other peoples' keto successes can be inspiring, but you don't see the struggles they experience getting to their successes. Also, every person responds differently to keto, and you have to find that balance within the diet that works for you. It's important to not compare yourself to others, so you avoid getting discouraged. So, with keto, you need to be more realistic with yourself and your goals, rather than overly strict.
2. **Take it slowly:** Losing quickly makes you feel great, but it's also not sustainable or healthy for you. Realistically, you should be aiming for 2lb / 1kg of weight loss per week. And don't climb on the scales too often either! Keep a record of a weekly weigh in and waist measurement and if you think it's going too slowly, change up the diet.
3. **Keep it Simple:** If you want to try your hand at the keto diet, keep it simple. Just keep reminding yourself that it's High-Fat and Low-Carb and you will see results.
4. **Eating out:** Just because you're on diet, doesn't mean you have to forego that birthday at a restaurant. Choose a meal that has meat or fish and change up the fries for extra veg. Have a burger without the buns. For dessert have a bowl of berries with some fresh cream.

5. **Clean out your Closet:** By that we mean your kitchen cupboard. Keeping treats in the kitchen will create temptations. While some days you will have the strength to say no, there will be days when you are not so motivated, and knowing that candy bar is in the back of the cupboard, will gnaw at you.

# EXCLUSIVE BONUS!

## Get Keto Audiobook for FREE NOW!*

***The Ultimate Keto Diet Guide 2019-2020:***
***How to Loose weight with Quick and Easy Steps***

SCAN ME

or go to

www.free-keto.co.uk

*Listen free for 30 Days on Audible (for new members only)

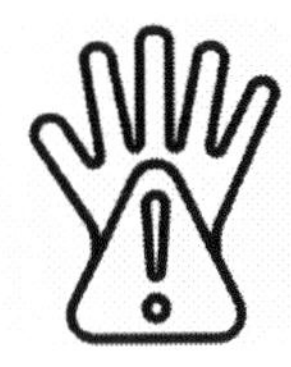

The opinions and ideas of the author contained in this publication are designed to educate the reader in an informative and helpful manner. While we accept that the instructions will not suit every reader, it is only to be expected that the recipes might not gel with everyone. Use the book responsibly and at your own risk. This work with all its contents, does not guarantee correctness, completion, quality or correctness of the provided information. Always check with your medical practitioner should you be unsure whether to follow a low carb eating plan. Misinformation or misprints cannot be completely eliminated. Human error is real!

Picture: zarzamora // shutterstock.com

Design: Oliviaprodesign

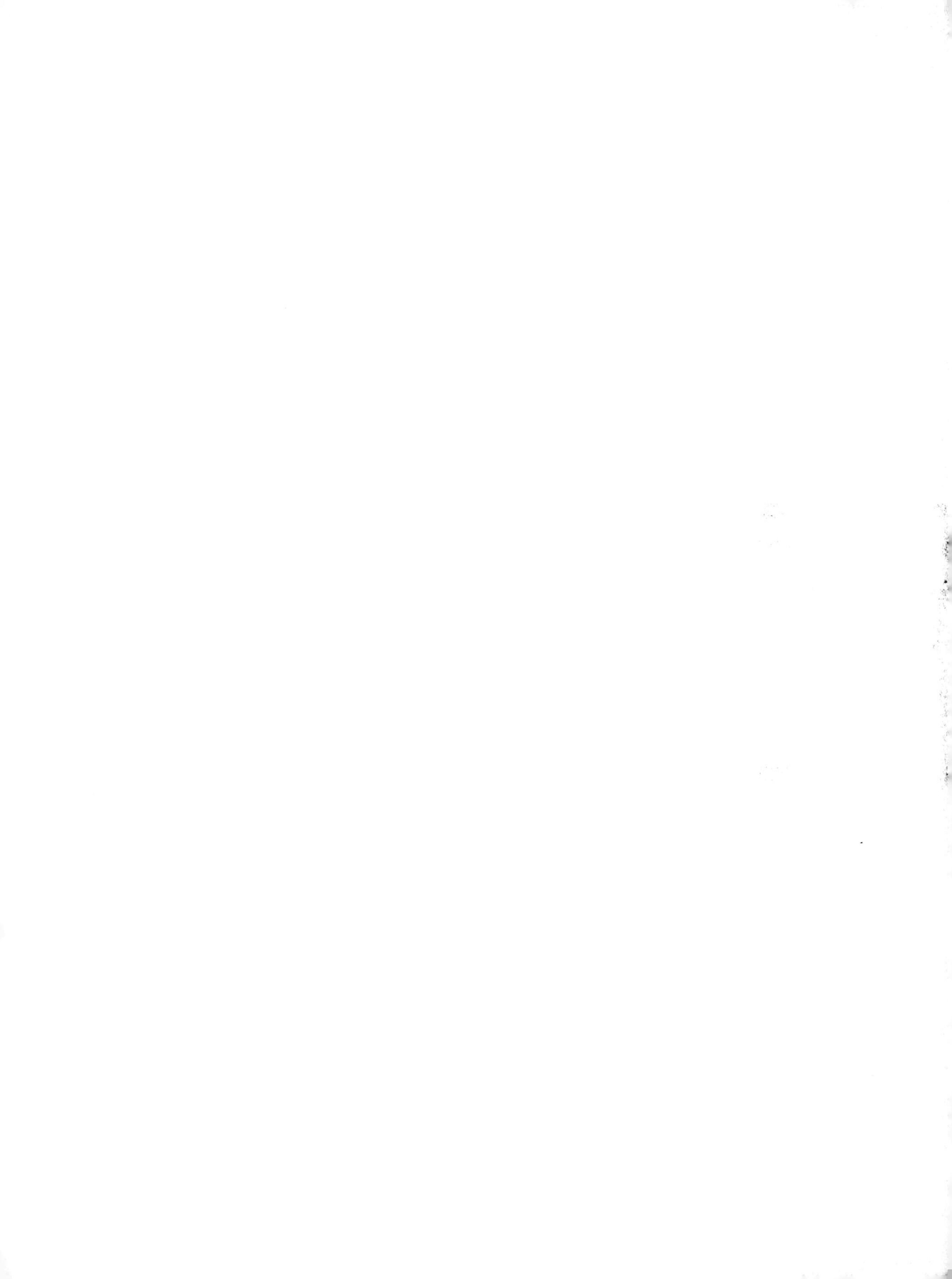

Printed in Great Britain
by Amazon